VITAMIN D RECEPTOR
GENE POLYMORPHISMS
AND
THE RISKS OF
BREAST CANCER

by

Ejike R. Egwuekwe

iUniverse books may be ordered through booksellers or by contacting:

iUniverse
1663 Liberty Drive
Bloomington, IN 47403
www.iuniverse.com
1-800-Authors (1-800-288-4677)

ISBN: 978-1-5320-9555-9 (sc)
ISBN: 978-1-5320-9556-6 (e)

Library of Congress Control Number: 2020903112

Print information available on the last page.

iUniverse rev. date: 02/18/2020

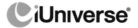

Disclaimer

The study of Medicine, its application in relation to curing of diseases, and the study of Epidemiology and its constitutive application to disease prevention and the minimization of disease exacerbation are evolutionary and continuously an ever-changing science. For these reasons, new researches are on-going, as clinical experiences keep broadening our knowledge base in ways and means to treat diseases, the types of drugs and vitamin supplements to apply in order to achieve better therapeutic outcomes. All these notwithstanding, the author of this book consulted with various sources believed to be reliable in an effort to provide data that are complete, unbiased, and in accord with acceptable standards at the time of this publication. Even though all these efforts were made to provide complete and (near) accurate information, the possibility still remains that human error may convey unintended meanings or outcomes to users of this piece of work. Furthermore, as indicated above, medical sciences and epidemiology are in constant evolution. Therefore, as things change or evolve, neither the author nor the publisher of this book guarantees that the data or information found herein is in every respect complete and accurate. For these reasons, I, the author disclaim every responsibility for any errors or omissions that may accrue from using any part of the information obtained from this book. Readers are encouraged to review other sources of information, and consult with their personal physicians before making health decisions. For example and very profoundly, readers are advised to consult with their personal physicians in cases when and if they see any abnormal growth or changes in their breasts and/or any body parts, rather than self-medicating or relying only on the information obtained from this book. Doing so would be a gross error and seriously contraindicated.

Abstract

Breast cancer is a world health problem and is a leading cause of cancer-related death among women in the United States. However, research has indicated that breast cancer risks could be reduced through exposure to Vitamin D by means of its Receptors identified as p53 target gene. The purpose of this research was to assess the associations between Vitamin D Receptor (VDR) gene polymorphisms (FokI and BsmI) and the risks of breast cancer among women. The research was carried out in Texas, USA. The research/study was guided by the theoretical framework of Roy adaptation model (RAM). The dependent variable was risk of breast cancer. The independent variables were knowledge about VDR gene polymorphisms and exposure to vitamin D. The relevant covariates considered in the research were the level of education, awareness, lifestyle, breast self-exams, mammograms, age, early menarche, late menopause, and family history of breast cancer among the participants. The chi-square test was used to test the stated research hypotheses and to answer the research questions. This research found that knowledge of VDR gene polymorphisms and exposure to vitamin D were not significantly associated with breast cancer risk, $\chi 2$ (3, N= 250) = 3.84, $p > 0.05$. Furthermore, this research found that awareness of the risk factors for breast cancer was not significantly associated with individuals' decisions to go for mammogram screenings or to enroll in breast cancer risk-reduction programs, $\chi 2$ (3, N= 250) =1.58, $p > 0.05$. To advocate for the promotion of awareness of the importance of pharmacogenetic testing for VDR gene polymorphisms for early detection of breast cancer, which would help to undertake appropriate therapeutic measures in a timely manner to prevent cancer metastasis, further research is warranted.

Vitamin D Receptor Gene Polymorphisms And Breast Cancer

by

Ejike R. Egwuekwe

Contents

List of Tables

List of Figures

Chapter 1: Introduction to the Study

Introduction

Breast cancer is a disease that affects men and women around the world; however, it occurs more often in women than in men. Although breast cancer occurs less frequently in men than in women, men with Klinefelter syndrome (47, XXY genotype) are 19-times more at risk for developing breast cancer than the general population of men without the syndrome. This is because males with Klinefelter syndrome have excessive estrogen stimulation in them. Nonetheless, in this research, my focus is on women's breast cancer rather than on men's. In the United States, more Caucasian American women are diagnosed with breast cancer each year than any other race or ethnicity (CDC, 2014). Although African American women are the second highest group of women diagnosed with breast cancer, they have a higher death rate from breast cancer than any other racial groups (American Cancer Society, 2015; CDC, 2016).

Breast cancer is idiopathic, and previous researchers do not understand the various risk factors for the disease. Some of the suspected risk factors for breast cancer include age, gender, environment, poor socioeconomic status, menstrual history, nulliparity, ethnicity, lifestyle (poor intake of vitamin D, either through direct exposure to sunlight or dietary supplements), and genetics, which includes mutations at p53, BRCA1, BRCA2, and in the Vitamin D Receptors. Previous researchers only focused on educational measures that emphasized using diet and exercise to reduce breast cancer risks (Guyton, Kensler, & Posner, 2003; Harvie et al., 2013). However, there had not been any epidemiologic study on the triangular association between Vitamin D metabolism, Vitamin D Receptor gene polymorphisms, and breast cancer risk at the individual level (John, Schwartz, Dreon, & Koo, 2011). Because Vitamin D Receptor gene polymorphisms had been implicated in breast cancers involving African American and Caucasian American women (Mishra et al., 2013), in this research, I assessed the level of knowledge and awareness of the target population in deficient areas in order to reduce breast cancer prevalence. Figure 1 reveals that breast cancer is more prevalent in Caucasian American women than in any other ethnic group.

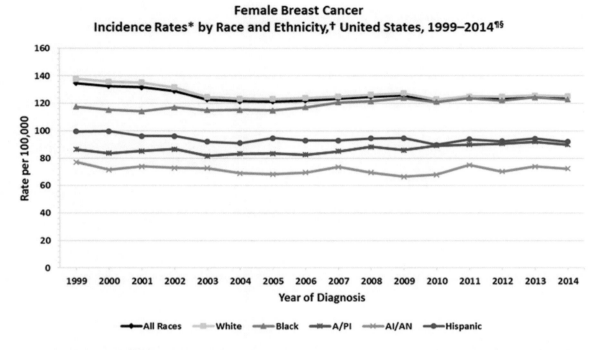

*Figure 1.*Incidence of breast cancer by ethnicity. Adapted from "Female Breast Cancer Incidence Rates by Race and Ethnicity, United States, 1999 to 2014." (cdc.gov/cancer/breast/statistics/race.htm)

Background of the Problem

According to the CDC (2014) and the Dana-Faber Cancer Institute (2017), breast cancer is the most commonly diagnosed form of all cancers among women in the United States. Jemal et al. (2014) reported that breast cancer is the second leading cancer-related death in the United States, second only to lung cancer. Vitamin D has been hypothesized as a potential cost-effective means of lowering the risk of breast cancer. However, a number of abnormal Vitamin D Receptors (in the Fok1, Bsm1, Apa1, Taq1, Calcitriol, and single nucleotide polymorphisms genes) are suspected to increase breast cancer incidence rates among African American and Caucasian American women, but not among Hispanic American, American Indian, or Asian American women.

Increasing the awareness of African American and Caucasian American women regarding breast cancer risk factors and the roles of Vitamin D Receptor gene polymorphisms in breast cancer may reduce breast cancer incidence among these ethnic groups. For example, it might motivate the subjects to adopt positive attitudes toward health and breast cancer screening and improve their intake of vitamin D. Furthermore, promoting knowledge in this area may reduce breast cancer incidence, which, according to Jemal et al. (2014), accounts for more than 25% of all cancer incidence rates (see Figure 2) and 15% of all cancer-related deaths among women in the United States (see Figure 3).

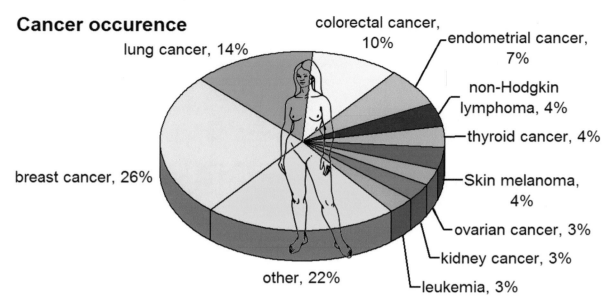

*Figure 2.*Cancer occurrence by percentage. Adapted from "Most Common Cancers—Female by Occurrence," by Jemal et al., 2014, *Cancer Journal for Clinicians,58*, pp. 71–96.

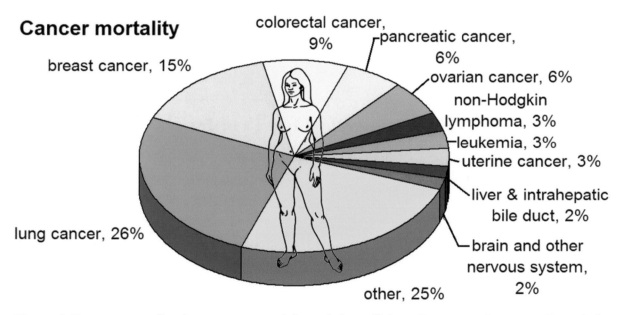

*Figure 3.*Cancer mortality by percentage. Adapted from "Most Common Cancers—Female by Occurrence," by Jemal et al., 2014, *Cancer Journal for Clinicians, 58,*pp. 71–96.

Problem Statement

Breast cancer is a health problem whose exact causes are unknown. It is the second leading cause of cancer-related deaths in the United States, second only to lung cancer (CDC, 2015; Grant, 2013). The U.S. National Breast Cancer Foundation (2015) and the American Cancer Society (2015, 2018) maintained that approximately one in eight women and one in 1,000 men would be diagnosed with breast cancer in their lifetime. Furthermore, in the United States, it was estimated that about 266,120 new cases of invasive breast cancer and 63,960 new cases of noninvasive (in situ) breast cancer would be diagnosed in women in 2018. The current estimates are higher than 2017 estimated diagnoses of about 252,710 cases of invasive and 63,410 cases of noninvasive breast cancers, respectively. The estimates should be checked every year, as the disease outlook changes from year to year. The exact causes of breast cancer are not known; because of this, only risk factors of breast cancer are usually discussed (Engel et al., 2011). Moreover, many African American women are unaware of the risk factors associated with breast cancer, especially in respect to genetic predisposition, ethnicity, and geographic regions of breast cancer prevalence (Mohr, Garland, Gorham, Grant, & Garland, 2008; National Cancer Foundation, 2015).

Scholars have indicated that, when compared with normal breast cells, breast cancer cells contain a lesser amount of Vitamin D Receptors (VDR). Abnormal or cancerous breast cells express abnormal Vitamin D Receptors than normal or noncancerous breast cells. This could be due to the polymorphisms induced by the VDR gene, and/or due to DNA methylation. Other researchers have focused only on disseminating information about using diet and exercise to reduce the risk factors of breast cancer (Guyton, Kensler, & Posner, 2003; Harvie et al., 2013).

John et al. (2011) maintained that there were no epidemiological studies on the relationship between Vitamin D metabolism and breast cancer risk at the individual level. Thus, promoting knowledge in this area became crucial, especially as the VDR gene polymorphisms have been associated with breast cancer in African Americans and Caucasian Americans, but not in Hispanic/Latina Americans. There might be a link between the VDR-FokI FF genotype and poor breast cancer prognoses among African American women diagnosed with breast cancer. These postulations left gaps in the literature worthy of further investigation. The investigation gave birth to this research.

Purpose of the Study

The purpose of this study was to assess the associations between Vitamin D and VDR gene polymorphisms and breast cancer risks among women in Dallas, Houston, and San Antonio, Texas, in the Southern United States.

Significance of the Study

The Fok1 gene is an essential Vitamin D Receptor that helps adequate metabolism of vitamin D. However, any mutation in this gene could produce two alleles or abnormal variants (VDRFF and VDRff) that may increase the risks of breast cancer (Guy et al., 2008; Knight, Lesosky, Barnett, Raboud, & Vieth,2007; Mishra et al., 2013; McGee, Durham, Tse, & Millikan, 2014). Although scholars have supported the possibilities of a link between VDR polymorphisms and increased breast cancer risks, no literature existed on the target population on the differences between Vitamin D and VDR to improve awareness in regard to the adverse effects of mutant VDRs. It therefore became necessary to conduct a research, and utilize the research findings to educate the target population, especially the African American women, about these risk factors and make them aware of the importance of genetic testing and breast cancer screenings.

A lack of awareness and poor socioeconomic status can reduce knowledge of the importance of genetic testing and breast cancer screenings. A lack of awareness can also lead to late cancer diagnoses and poor prognoses. According to the American Cancer Society (2013), and the CDC (2016), African American women have lower rates of mammographic screenings than Caucasian American women and Hispanic American women. This could be a reason for the high incidence of breast cancer morbidity and mortality prevalence among African American women.

The results obtained from this research could have positive social change implications black (African American) women in particular and women in general. For example, the research/study could promote awareness among the target population regarding the importance of participating in regular breast cancer screenings. The study could also increase the awareness of the at-risk population in respect to pharmacogenetic testing for VDR gene polymorphisms capable of causing breast cancer. There have not been epidemiological studies on the triangular associations between Vitamin D metabolism, VDR polymorphisms, and breast cancer risks at the level of the target population. Therefore, this research/study could promote awareness at the individual level. Promoting awareness and understanding of the importance of breast cancer screening among African American and Caucasian American women could lead to early cancer detection among this group of women.

Additionally, the research/study could improve the understanding of the importance of adequate Vitamin D intake. Vitamin D can be obtained either through direct sunlight or through dietary supplements. Accessing Vitamin D through dietary means is important for those who do not have adequate sun exposure due to religious, medical, or other personal reasons. Furthermore, the outcomes of this research could be helpful to clinicians in formulating effective therapies and treatment regimens to increase the rate of Vitamin D absorption, especially among African American women, whose thick skins make it difficult to absorb and metabolize sufficient Vitamin D through ambient sources. Finally, the intervention protocols addressed in this study may promote participation in programs that may reduce breast cancer morbidity and mortality rates among African American and Caucasian American women. For example, as shown in Figure 4, only 17% of African American women participate in regular mammograms.

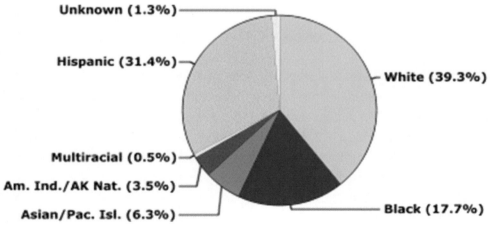

Figure 4. Five-year summary of mammograms: January 2011 to December 2015.Adapted from "Breast Cancer Screening." (cdc.gov/cancer/nbccedp/data/summaries/national aggregate.htm)

Theoretical Framework

The Roy adaptation model (RAM) was used to guide this study. Since 1976, when the theory was developed, it has been used in various nursing and public health situations to overcome life-threatening circumstances. The theory was applied to increase participation of adults and ailing populations in age-appropriate physical activity (PA) programs and to improve the health and physical well-being of participants in various programs listed in *Healthy People 2010* (CDC, 2011).The primary concern of the elderly is the decline in their physical functions. This is usually compounded with challenges in health resulting from an increased prevalence of sedentary lifestyle (Nelson et al., 2007). RAM emphasizes the importance of behavioral change through the use of interventions such as physical activities to promote adaptation to the aging process and to minimize the disease process among older adults (La Forge, 2005).

The RAM has also been used in holistic oncology practice to assess the behaviors of breast cancer patients and to evaluate the stimuli influencing their behavioral change (Piazza, Foote, Holcombe, Harris, & Wright, 2007). It is necessary to assess whether individual risk behaviors such as lack of exposure to sunlight or vitamin D, low level of education, breast self-examinations, mammograms, cigarette smoking, poor nutritional intake, and sedentary lifestyle might be contributory factors in breast cancer exacerbation.

Furthermore, RAM has been applied in programs associated with resilience. The American College of Sports Medicine (ACSM, 2005) and the American Heart Association (AHA, 2007) revealed that 47% of adults 65 to 74 years of age, and 60% of adults 75 years of age and older were not active in any leisure time activities. These data were an indication that the aging population was falling short of the *Healthy People 2010* goals and the ACSM and AHA guidelines on physical activity for older adults. The RAM was then used to get older adults to enroll in physical activity programs to meet the recommended guideline of about 30 minutes of moderate intensity physical activity at least five times a week. It was also applied in strength training with balance and flexibility training two times per week, as recommended (Beaudreau, 2006).

The RAM includes the term environment as all conditions, circumstances, and influences that surround and affect the development and behavior of an individual person (Rogers & Keller, 2009). The theory also sees everyone as a biopsychosocial being or a set of interrelated beings comprising biological, psychological, and social interplay in constant interaction with a changing environment in which the individual strives to live within a unique band as he or she tries to cope with a given situation (Young-McCaughan et al., 2007). The RAM employs three stressors, which include *focal stimulus, contextual stimulus,* and *residual stimulus.* Focal stimuli include any illness or problems immediately confronting the individual in any situation (Rogers & Keller, 2009). They may also include immediate family needs, the level of family adaptation, and changes involving family members living within the same environment (Rogers & Keller, 2009). Contextual stimuli include anything that influences the situation (Rogers & Keller, 2009). Residual stimuli include things such as beliefs or attitudes that resonate from the person and are capable of influencing the situation. These may also include all the incidentals of unknown etiologies impacting the person at any given time (Rogers &Keller, 2009). A person is able to adapt to a negative situation depending on his or her abilities to manage the three stimuli.

In this study, the RAM was used to assess response efficacy in respect to perceived susceptibility to breast cancer and the perceived seriousness of engaging in health-promoting behaviors. RAM mirrors the health belief model in some areas. As revealed in Figure 5, people are likely to engage in health-promoting behaviors if the perceived benefits outweigh perceived disadvantages or barriers. This notion is shared in RAM, in which people are likely to enroll in programs that promote quality of life if the perceived advantage could lead to actions that reduce breast cancer risks.

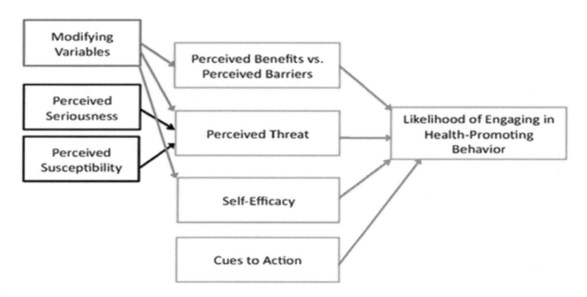

*Figure 5.*Modifying variables used in HBM and RAM on perceptions and attitudes of people toward benefits or barriers associated with health-promoting behaviors. Adapted from *Images for Health Belief Model*, by Jones & Bartlett Learning (2016). (www.jblearning.com/ samples/0763743836/)

Research Questions and Hypotheses

The following research questions were addressed in this study:

1. Is there an association between VDR gene polymorphisms knowledge/awareness and decisions to reduce breast cancer risks?

$H_0 1$: There is no association between VDR gene polymorphisms knowledge/awareness and decisions to reduce breast cancer risks.

$H_a 1$: There is an association between VDR gene polymorphisms knowledge/awareness and decisions to reduce breast cancer risks.

2. Is there an association between knowledge of VDR gene polymorphisms and likelihood of mammogram screening?

$H_0 2$: There is no association between knowledge of VDR gene polymorphisms and likelihood of mammogram screening.

$H_a 2$: There is an association between knowledge of VDR gene polymorphisms and likelihood of mammogram screening.

Nature of the Study

This was a quantitative research study. It used a quasi-experimental approach to determine the efficacies of programs that participants used in reducing breast cancer risks. Levels of awareness regarding the impacts of vitamin D Receptor gene polymorphisms in increasing breast cancer risks were assessed. I also assessed whether or not the subjects' involvements in breast cancer risk-reduction programs were effective. Using a quantitative design was necessary. It helped in maintaining consistency for data presentation, especially when documenting and analyzing data differentiating the various effects of VDR gene polymorphisms on African American and Caucasian American women. The design also proved helpful when assessing and documenting the effectiveness of the subjects' program involvement to maintain resilience, self-efficacy, genetic testing, and mammographic screenings.

Definitions of Terms

The following terms were used throughout the study:

Breast cancer: A malignant growth that starts when a breast cell, with damaged DNA begins to grow out of control and invade other body tissues (American Cancer Society, 2013).

Deoxyribonucleic acid (DNA): A molecule that encodes all genetic instructions used in the functioning of living organisms and viruses (Haga & LaPointe, 2013; Ohanuka, 2017).

Effect: Outcome, result, consequence.

International unit (IU): Universally used in measuring biological activities of vitamin D. For example, 1 unit of IU is equivalent to 0.025 micrograms cholecalciferol, ergocalciferol, and 1,25dihydroxyvitamin D_3 all of which are different forms of vitamin (Buhler, 1988, 2001).

Environment: An area or a surrounding, state, city, town, or village in which people live. Such people are breathing the same type of air, having the same amount of sunlight, eating the same or similar types of food, and having access to the same types of Vitamin D supplements.

Hypervitaminosis D: High serum vitamin D.

Hypovitaminosis D: Low metabolism of vitamin D.

Delimitations

This study was based on a sample size of 250 women. The sample size was selected from three Texas cities (Dallas, Houston, and San Antonio). Although the population was randomly selected from among these populous cities, it cannot be seen as a true representation of the entire Southern United States, nor can it be held as a true representation of the entire state of Texas. However, this was the least costly approach that could be undertaken and still be able to satisfy the research purpose and objectivity. Furthermore, I cannot claim that the results of this study are complete. I also cannot claim to hold all the answers to breast cancer risks.

According to the CDC (2014), the incidence rates of breast cancer vary by ethnicity and geographic location. Although the three chosen cities are all in Texas, a Southern U. S. state, levels of sunlight in these cities vary according to latitude and geographical climatic conditions. For example, Houston is hotter than San Antonio and Dallas, and San Antonio is hotter than Dallas. Thus, the participants could not be said to receive the same level of sunlight exposure, even though the length of exposures could be similar. Furthermore, by focusing only on these three cities, other geographic areas in the Southern United States, and the entire United States in general, were left unassessed. In addition, comorbidities that could have precipitated malignant breast tumors might have been left undiscussed, as they were outside the scope of this research.

Limitations

SurveyMonkey approach was used in recruiting participants for this study. For example, survey materials were distributed and/or mailed out to individual participants. One problem with this approach was that it was not certain that someone other than the respondent filled out the questionnaire on behalf of that particular respondent. Furthermore, there was no way of verifying the accuracy of information or data supplied by the respondents. For example, a person could have denied personal or family history of breast cancer, when the contrary was the case. Additionally, a person could have been inaccurate in reporting extents of involvement with breast self-examinations, mammogram screenings, exposure to sunlight, and Vitamin

D intake. Furthermore, as this study included individuals older than 65 years, it was possible that some individuals may have forgotten the age at which they observed their menarche or first menstrual flow. Any recall bias and/or inaccurate reporting could distort the internal and external validities of this research.

Assumptions

Vitamin D intake was assumed to be a factor in reducing the risk of breast cancer. It was further assumed that insufficiency in Vitamin D (i.e., hypovitaminosis D) affects about 50% of the world's population, due to lifestyle (reduced outdoor activities and wearing of certain protective religious garments), and environmental reasons (air pollution). A combination of these factors could be assumed to have led to reduced exposure to ambient sunlight, an important source of Vitamin D.

It was also assumed that individuals who were sensitive to sunlight exposure, or individuals suffering from photophobia, due to any number of reasons, did not participate in this research. It was further assumed that individuals allergic to supplemental or dietary Vitamin D were excluded from this study. Inclusion of respondents who did not meet inclusion criteria could negatively impact the external and internal validities of this study. It was assumed that all participants were capable of having adequate exposures to daily intake of Vitamin D through direct sunlight or supplements. Additionally, it was assumed that women deficient in Vitamin D adhered to the prescribed treatment regimens with either vitamin D_2 or vitamin D_3 and other required programs that could help in reducing breast cancer risks and prevalence, thus reducing mortality from the disease.

Possible Types and Sources of Information or Data

The study utilized data extracted from the Texas Cancer Registry. Some other valuable data were obtained through direct conversations and interviews with directors of breast cancer treatment centers and hospitals, among other sources. This quasi-experimental study examined a sample size of 250 individuals, which included 125 cases and 125 controls. Both arms contained premenopausal and postmenopausal women.

SurveyMonkey approach was used in distributing survey questionnaires. This method was also used in recruiting and interviewing participants about their knowledge concerning the differences between vitamin D, VDRs, the negative impacts of VDR polymorphisms with respect to breast cancer, and their knowledge about the importance of using exposure to Vitamin D and mammograms to reduce the risk of developing breast cancer.

Summary

Breast cancer is a disease of unknown etiology in which malignant (cancer) cells form in the tissues of the breast. While it can occur in both men and women, the vast majority (99%) of cases occur in women. It is the most common cancer in women globally. According to the American Cancer Society (2010), each year about 1.3 million women are diagnosed with breast cancer worldwide, and more than 465,000 die from the disease each year. Breast cancer is the leading killer of women aged 20 to 59 worldwide (World Health Organization, 2013). Twenty-five percent of women diagnosed with breast cancer die within 5 years, and 40% die within 10 years of their diagnosis (American Cancer Society, 2017). Breast cancer in younger women (under age 50) tends to be more aggressive and more malignant (Carolinathermascan, 2013). The increase in morbidity and mortality rates accruing from this disease has produced the need for further research. Although some attempts were previously made toward identifying the association between VDR gene polymorphisms and the prognosis for breast cancer, the findings were inconclusive. Thus, further research was warranted.

The lack of Vitamin D has been associated with a risk of breast cancer development. An abundance of exposure to Vitamin D could play a role in (breast) cancer risk reduction. The disease risk could further be reduced through supplemental Vitamin D therapies. For instance, adequate Vitamin D supplementation could work with the genetic factor of VDR by bolstering the presence of Vitamin D in serum through metabolism and by its availability in human cells. Vitamin D is a fat-soluble prohormone that can be modified within the body to produce and promote some active metabolites.

There are two types of vitamin D: vitamin D_2 and vitamin D_3. Vitamin D_2, or ergocalciferol, is derived from plants or vegetation. On the other hand, vitamin D_3, or cholecalciferol or 7-dehydrocholesterol, is metabolized in human skin and is derived from exposure to ultraviolet B (UVB) light emanating from the sun. Vitamin D_3 has also been identified in certain foods of animal origin (i.e., egg yolks, dairy fats, liver, and oily fish). These sources, however, offer a modest 10% amount of vitamin D, while the majority (up to 90%) of Vitamin D is derived from endogenous production in the human skin.

African Americans have the lowest levels of serum vitamin D. This is because darker skins do not easily absorb and/or metabolize vitamin D from sunlight. Therefore, VDR haplotypes are associated with breast cancer among African American women, but not in Hispanic women. Furthermore, the VDR-FokI FF genotype has been linked with poor prognoses in African American women diagnosed with breast cancer. These reasons, in addition to inaccessibility to healthcare, could account for why more African American women die from the disease than other races or ethnicities. However, this ethnic group could benefit from information regarding VDR gene polymorphisms. Thus, I examined whether knowledge/awareness of VDR gene polymorphisms' association with breast cancer could increase participants' desire to go for mammograms and reduce the risks associated with breast cancer.

In the United States, more Caucasian American women are diagnosed with breast cancer than any other race or ethnicity. However, African American women have the highest death rate from breast cancer than any other ethnic group. Although previous researchers have discussed various risk factors associated with breast cancer, John et al. (2011) revealed that there have not been any epidemiologic studies on the relationship between Vitamin D metabolism and breast cancer risks at the individual level. It therefore became imperative to research and promote knowledge in this area.

There are some positive social change implications that could be derived from this research. For example, an increased awareness of the associations between Vitamin D metabolism, VDR gene polymorphisms, and breast cancer risks could motivate concerned individuals to take necessary steps to reduce breast cancer risks.

In Chapter 2, I present the literature review for this study. I also discuss issues pertaining to increased awareness of breast cancer screening methods, including the importance of breast self-examination and clinical breast examination (or mammograms) and the impacts of VDR gene polymorphisms.

Chapter 2: Literature Review

Introduction

In this chapter, issues regarding awareness and the importance of breast cancer screening through breast self-examination and clinical breast examination (i.e., mammogram) are discussed. Its focus is on the impact of VDR gene polymorphisms and the risks of breast cancer among women in Texas, in the Southern United States. The chapter begins with the literature search strategy, after which a review of methods is discussed. Next, the studies related to the method, before discussing the studies related to the content, are discussed. Tables are used, where applicable, to illustrate the levels of awareness, knowledge, behaviors, and attitudes of women toward Vitamin D intake and breast cancer screening as strategies for reducing breast cancer risks. The literature related to the study and threats to the validity of the study are also discussed in this chapter. The other topics discussed in this chapter include breast cancer preview, the risk factors for breast cancer, the role of mammogram and breast self-exams, and the role of VDR gene polymorphisms in cancer risks. Also discussed in this chapter are the roles of Vitamin D and sunlight exposure in breast cancer prevention, the overview of RAM, and the importance of knowledge in reducing breast cancer risks.

Literature Search Strategy

To search for relevant materials suitable for this study, several search engines and databases were used, including PubMed, MEDLINE, EMBASE, Scopus, Web of Science, the Google Scholar, CNKI, CINAHL, CBM, and the American Society of Clinical Oncology. The key words used were *VDR gene polymorphisms and breast cancer risks, association between VDR gene polymorphisms and breast cancer risks, the association between Fok1,Bsm1, Apa1, Taq1 or poly-A repeat polymorphisms of the VDR gene and breast cancer risk, abnormal Fok1 and breast cancer, Fok1 variants VDRff and VDRFF, female reproductive cancers and genetics, genetic bases of female reproductive cancers, mammalian epithelial cancers and Fok1 gene, Fok1 oncogenes and female mammary gland,* and *single nucleotide polymorphisms (SNPs) or SNP and breast cancer.* However, most of the data used in this study were obtained from women that participated in the research and from the Texas Cancer Registry.

Data were also obtained from articles in the American Cancer Society (2013), Susan G. Komen (2015), and the CDC (2016) that discussed African American and Caucasian American women's levels of awareness in the use of Vitamin D (either through direct exposure to sunlight or through dietary supplement) in reducing breast cancer risks. Peer-reviewed and non-peer-reviewed articles were used in this study. Attempts were also made to collect and compare breast cancer data or information from hospital records. Two major hospitals (M. D. Anderson Cancer Treatment Center in Houston, Texas and Southwestern University Medical Center – Cancer Unit in Dallas, Texas) and a cancer treatment facility in Dallas, Texas were consulted.

Survey materials were distributed to, and collected from, the participants using a SurveyMonkey method. In the survey questions, I focused on the subjects' knowledge about the differences between Vitamin D and VDR. I also asked about the negative impacts of VDR gene polymorphisms in relation to breast cancer. The subjects' knowledge about Vitamin D Receptor polymorphisms and the importance of using Vitamin D to reduce their chances of getting breast cancer were also addressed through the survey. Finally, I asked questions about the participants' knowledge in respect to using regular breast exams in early cancer detection.

This was a case-control study with a sample size of 250. It contained 125 women in the case group and 125 women in the control group. Of these, 75 women in the control group were premenopausal, while the other 75 in the case group were postmenopausal. The premenopausal category consisted of women (<45 years of age) and the postmenopausal category comprised women (>45 years of age).

Review of Methods

The scholars represented in this literature review used the quantitative research approach. The quantitative research approach is measurable and was better suited to determine the effectiveness of the programs that participants used while attempting to reduce breast cancer risks. Thus, the quantitative research method became a useful tool in assessing subjects' knowledge and levels of awareness regarding the impacts of VDR gene polymorphisms in breast cancer risks. Furthermore, this method was adopted in order to guide consistency in data presentation. This could be crucial, especially when documenting and analyzing data. Additionally, the quantitative method was the most appropriate approach for this study, especially when testing the theories and when predicting program outcomes.

The RAM theoretical concept, which has applicability in health behavior changes, was used in this study. Evaluating levels of behavior changes among participants in breast cancer research was more quantitative than qualitative. This was another reason for adopting this method. Because participants in this research were randomly recruited through SurveyMonkey approach, and because the cancer rates were extrapolated from cancer statistics from state cancer registries, this was a quasi-experimental study.

Studies Related to the Method

The United States Preventive Services Task Force (USPSTF) recommended that women whose family histories suggest increased risk of hereditary breast or ovarian cancer (HBOC) be referred for genetic counseling (Chen & Li, 2015). African American and Hispanic American women in the United States are more likely to be diagnosed with late-stage breast cancer and are less likely to survive the disease. However, more African American and Caucasian American women die from the disease than women from any other race or ethnicity (see Figure 6).

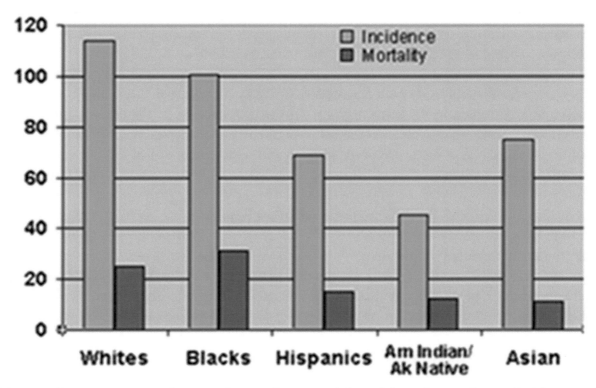

Figure 6. Breast cancer incidence and mortality rates. Adapted from *Breast Cancer Incidence and Mortality Rates by Race (2008 to 2012) Surveillance, Epidemiology, and End Result Program*, by National Cancer Institute, 2015. (https://breast-cancer.ca/mort-racing/)

In order to implement the USPSTF guidelines, there is a need to obtain family histories of hereditary breast and ovarian cancers. Therefore, feasible methods have to be employed for family history risk assessment. For example, in an assessment to study the possibility of using a self-administered web-based survey to collect personal and family histories of cancer, it was found that 28% of the women were considered appropriate for genetic counseling. The ease of a self-administered web-based survey was the principal reason I decided to use this method. Thus, based on the successes derived from such method, I considered a self-administered web-based survey as the most appropriate method for selecting subjects for cancer-related studies (or researches) and assessments.

In another development, an assessment of knowledge about breast cancer and screening methods was conducted among 281 Ethiopian nurses; and it was found that only 156 (57.8%) of the nurses were knowledgeable about breast cancer and mammographic screening and that 114 (42.2%) knew nothing about breast cancer (Lemlem et al, 2011). It therefore became apparent that the knowledge of this group of women was not satisfactory and that there was a need to improve the content of school curricula in order to improve women's knowledge in breast cancer and screening methods.

Similarly, a research was conducted to assess the awareness, knowledge, and attitudes of 373 Pakistani women toward breast cancer and early detection. The study revealed a general hesitation among Pakistani women to participate in breast cancer research. It was thereby observed that Pakistani women did not like giving responses to questions related to their breasts or other parts of the body they considered sensitive, provocative, and embarrassing due to cultural stigma and societal conservatism. To circumnavigate through such obstacle, Naqvi, Zehra, Ahmad, and Ahmad (2016) developed a breast cancer inventory (BCI) method that used web-based self-administered surveys, which was successfully used to assess the Pakistani women's awareness, knowledge, and attitudes regarding breast cancer and early detection techniques.

Given the level of success achieved through the method of administering surveys and gathering sensitive health data from subjects, providing access to this type of tool at the time of mammography could make women embrace clinical breast exams without shyness, bashfulness, or embarrassment. Therefore, successfully using this approach could increase the feasibility of identifying and referring women for genetic consultation regarding hereditary breast-ovarian cancer susceptibility. This was another good reason for my adopting this method in administering the survey material.

It is notable that in 2016, the Planned Parenthood Federation of America used a nationwide survey to explore women's experiences, knowledge, and beliefs about cervical and breast cancer screenings. Similarly, a survey was used to assess the barriers women experienced in accessing preventive care. Furthermore, through a survey, the Planned Parenthood Federation of America was able to find out that differences existed among African American women, Hispanic American, and Caucasian American women, in terms of the barriers to getting screened for breast and cervical cancers. Although 73% of the women said that they understood how often women should be screened for cervical cancer, only 9% correctly answered that, on average, women between 21 and 29 years of age should be screened for cervical cancer every 3 years, and that women between the ages of 30–64 should be screened for cervical cancer every 3–5 years. Although most (84%) of the women said they understood how often they should be screened for breast cancer, only 10% correctly answered that on average, women between 21–39 years old should be screened for breast cancer every 1–3 years, depending on personal and family history. McDonald-Mosley of the Planned Parenthood Federation of America revealed that 23% of the women indicated that they did not know when they should next go for breast cancer screening, and 39% of women stated that they did not know when next to go for cervical cancer screening. Similarly, 32% of African American women and 42% of Hispanic American women saw cost as a barrier to breast and cervical cancer screening, compared to 19% of Caucasian American women (Planned Parenthood Federation of America, 2016).

In an assessment about sources of Vitamin D conducted among 915 young Korean breast cancer survivors and 29,694 controls (i.e., those without a history of cancer) and those who worked indoors, the women were analyzed as to whether they were predisposed to Vitamin D deficiency. The women's serum Vitamin D levels were measured, and individuals with 25(OH)D levels less than 20 ng/mL were defined as deficient. By using survey method to obtain valuable data on breast cancer, it was found that inadequate exposures to Vitamin D were associated with poor breast cancer prognoses. Even though data in regard to actual Vitamin D levels among the breast cancer survivors were limited, it was possible to infer and thereby conclude that regular evaluation and management of Vitamin D levels were needed among Korean women (Oh et al, 2015). Survey, therefore, could play a positive role in obtaining breast cancer data. This substantiates another reason why I chose to use surveys in this breast cancer research.

Studies Related to the Content

Early detection is of importance in breast cancer treatment, cure, and survival rate. More than 90% of women diagnosed with breast cancer at an early stage survive the disease for 5 or more years, compared to only 15% of women diagnosed at advanced stages of the disease (Cancer Research UK, 2015). However, early diagnosis must be accompanied by ensuring that the patient receives the most effective and appropriate treatment regimens, without which the cancer may spread. There are five possible causes for late breast cancer diagnosis:

- Lack of knowledge and/or awareness of signs and symptoms of breast cancer
- The individual might be worried about what the doctor might find out
- Fear that husband, boyfriend, or significant other would leave, if breast cancer is diagnosed
- The primary care physician might have delayed referring patients for treatment
- Hospitals might have delayed giving the individuals appointments

In any of these scenarios, the cancer would continue to metastasize. Low level of knowledge and/or awareness of the importance of early breast cancer detection is of monumental repercussion and needs paramount redressing. For example, in a research on breast cancer early detection conducted among 7,066 Indian women aged 15–70, the women showed a varied level of awareness on the risk factors associated with breast cancer (i.e., family history (13–58%), reproductive history (1–88%), and obesity (11–51%). Although on average nurses are more aware of breast cancer incidence than the general population, in India, Indian nurses' knowledge and levels of awareness for risk factors of breast cancer were poor and grossly deficient. For example, in a research conducted over an 8-year period (2005–2013), there were poor literacy levels among Indian nurses in respect to risk factors of breast cancer. In another instance, about 40.8–98% of the Indian nurses who were surveyed were deemed deficient in knowledge and awareness about the association between family history and breast cancer. For example, about 21–90% knew nothing about the link between reproductive history and breast cancer; also, about 34–65% revealed no knowledge about any association between obesity and breast cancer (Gupta et al, 2015). It can therefore be stated without equivocation that low literacy in regard to breast cancer risk factors existed and still exist among Indian women, irrespective of their socioeconomic and educational background.

Poor knowledge and lack of awareness of breast cancer risk factors may lead to a delay in screening. A delay in screening may lead to a delay in diagnosis, which may lead to poor prognosis and rising incidence in mortality rates. Multiple stakeholders need to champion the course for the interest of society and the health system to cultivate and improve cancer literacy among women. This clarion call should resoundingly be heeded to, not only in the United States of America, Pakistan, or India, but around the world.

A research was conducted involving 17 regional churches in Chicago to verify whether faith-based approaches could be used to bridge racial and ethnic disparities in breast cancer screening programs. It was noted that African American and Hispanic American women consider the church as an influence in their cultural and community life. For this reason, inductions about mammographic screenings could be entrenched in church programs involving these ethnic groups. Such inductions could be instrumental among African Americans, Afro Caribbeans, and Nigerians, especially those who believe in miracle healings. The knowledge and awareness would enable miracle-seekers to add active therapeutic regimens to their repertoire.

In the University of Ibadan, Nigeria, 278 postgraduate female students were assessed in regards to their levels of awareness, knowledge, and practices regarding breast cancer screening. It was found that breast cancer burden is on the increase in Nigeria and that most cases present to hospitals at late stages, when cure has become elusive. The assessment also revealed that most of the postgraduate students indicated that they were knowledgeable about breast self-examination (BSE), clinical breast examination, and mammography. However, of the 159 participants who claimed to be practicing BSE, only 118 (58.4%) stated that they practiced it occasionally. Additionally, of the 53 postgraduate students who indicated that they had experienced clinical breast examination, only 7.4% had it performed on them by nurses or midwives. Furthermore, the study found that only 11.4% of the postgraduate students actually had good knowledge of BSEs. Similarly, among the postgraduate students, only 33.7% had good knowledge of breast cancer risk factors (Aluko et al, 2014).

To minimize deficits in knowledge in respect to breast cancer morbidity and risk factors, health workers should reach out to academic communities, either through cancer awareness programs, or through continuing education classes, or through adult education programs that could improve their knowledge about the disease. Taking this step could help impart in women effective breast cancer prevention practices. Both printed and electronic media are recommended to be used in disseminating health education material or information, to ensure wider coverage.

A cross-sectional study and self-administered questionnaires were used to assess the level of knowledge and awareness of breast cancer among 595 Angolan medical and nonmedical female university students. It was found that the majority of the Angolan women, including the medical students, were deficient in knowledge concerning symptoms of breast cancer, breast cancer risk factors, preventive measures in relation to breast cancer, and mammographic screenings (Sambanje and Mafuvadze, 2012). These findings were in accord with the extrapolations made from an assessment in regard to awareness, knowledge, and attitudes toward breast cancer and early detection conducted among Pakistani women, from which it was observed that Pakistani women knew little or nothing about breast cancer. From a cultural perspective, Pakistani women are generally hesitant to give responses in surveys related to breast cancer (Naqvi et al., 2016). This might be due to stigma and cultural conservatism among this group of women.

All in all, the majority of the participants in this research did not know anything about the early signs of breast cancer, such as change in color or shape of the nipple. Furthermore, majority of the people had no knowledge that individuals with dark skin pigmentation require more exposure to ambient sunlight to produce adequate vitamin D. Both in this research and in previous researches, while a number of the medical students claimed that they knew about breast self-examinations, very few actually practiced it.

Lack of knowledge and low awareness in respect to symptoms of breast cancer and breast cancer screening techniques are the probable causes of high breast cancer mortality rates among African Americans, Afro Caribbeans, and Sub-Saharan Africans. The need for increased breast cancer awareness among these ethnicities (as well as among Latina and Caucasian women) should be appreciated. This could be achieved through the help of departments of health and various applicable health organizations. Furthermore, breast cancer awareness could be entrenched in school curricula. This could be achieved by formulating health education programs that bolster breast cancer awareness, promote knowledge of screening techniques and the importance of early detection of breast cancer among women.

Literature Related to the Study

Although various studies assessing the associations between VDR gene polymorphisms and breast cancer risks often show controversial results, it has been hypothesized that VDR gene polymorphisms may influence both the risk of cancer occurrence and prognosis (Köstner et al., 2009). In a study conducted by Mishra et al. (2013), blood was drawn from 232 African American breast cancer patients (cases) and 349 non-cancer subjects. The study found a significant association between the VDR-Fok1*f*allele and breast cancer among African American women (OR=1.9, p=0.07). The research also found increased chances of breast cancer development among Latinas who carry the VDR-ApaI alleles (*Aa* or *aa*) (p=0.008).

In another research conducted among 230 Egyptian women (with 130 participants in the cases category aged 49 to 65, and 100 participants in the controls category aged 50 to 72), it was found that the BsmI bb and the ApaI aa genotypes were associated with significantly increased risks of breast cancer, while no significant associations were reported for the genotypes and allele frequencies of FokI and TaqI polymorphisms among these black women (Abd-Elsalam et al., 2015).

However, in two research studies involving 718 (255 cases/463 controls) and 1,596 (622 cases/974 controls) respectively, the *Fok*I and *Bsm*I genotypes among Caucasian women were analyzed. It was found that no statistically significant association existed between the two polymorphisms and breast cancer risks among Caucasian women (Sinotte et al., 2008).

Another research was conducted to determine the association between the VDR-FokI and BsmI polymorphisms among Iranian breast cancer patients. The case-control study involved 296 women, of which 140 were breast cancer patients, and 156 women were control. The research found a significantly increased risk of breast cancer with the BsmI bb (and the Bb) genotypes (with OR 2.39, CI 1.17-4.85, and OR 2.28, CI 1.16-4.47, respectively). However, no significant association was found between the FokI polymorphisms and breast cancer risk among this ethnic population (Uitterlindenet al., 2004; Shahbazi et al., 2013).

In a retrospective case-control study involving Caucasian women breast cancer patients (n = 398 cases and n = 427 controls), the risk factors of three VDR gene polymorphisms were analyzed. It was found that there was an association between VDR gene polymorphisms and breast cancer risk, and that it can influence breast cancer progression and metastasis. Additionally, in a case-control study on 296 Iranian women, among whom were 140 breast cancer patients and 156 age-matched control women, *Restriction fragment length polymorphisms* (RFLPs) analyses were performed for BsmI and FokI genotypes. The polymerase chain reaction (PCR) was randomly selected and the products were subjected to sequencing to verify the restriction fragment length polymorphism (RFLP) results. An increased risk of breast cancer was associated with the VDR-BsmI polymorphism in Iranian women; but no significant risk was associated with the VDR-FokI genotype among these women. On the contrary, in a nurse's health study conducted among African American women in the Southern United States, the genotypes of 1,234 incident cases and 1,676 controls for VDR-FokI, and 1,180 incident cases and 1,547 controls for VDR BsmI were analyzed. The research indicated that African American women with the ff genotype were more susceptible to breast cancer than people with the FF genotype (Chen et al., 2005).

Some meta-analyses by Tang et al. (2009) combined data sets extrapolated from 21 case studies encompassing more than 5,000 breast cancer cases. These meta-analyses provided evidence supporting a positive correlation between the VDR Fokl ff genotype and an amplified susceptibility to proliferative breast pathogenesis. Similarly, a large cohort study comprising 8,100 controls and 6,300 cases by McKay et al. (2009) affirmed the results of the meta-analysis. Additionally, the study supports the claim that the ff genotype is capable of augmenting the risk factor for breast cancer among African American women.

On the contrary, Abbas et al. (2008) found no correlation between the Fokl polymorphism and increase in breast cancer risk among postmenopausal Caucasian women. Similarly, in a meta-analysis comprising eight prospective nested case-control studies, Lu, Jing, and Zhang (2016) found no association between VDR gene polymorphism (Fok1) and breast cancer in the Caucasian ethnic subgroup.

Put together, the inconsistencies in these research findings were ample indications that additional investigations were required to know how different genotypes affect the functional mechanisms of Vitamin D Receptors (VDRs) in the breast cells of various ethnic groups. It then became an area to be explored in this research. Knowing this could provide a better insight and strategy for identifying women at risk of breast cancer. The knowledge, insight, and strategy may in turn be helpful in developing improved breast cancer treatment regimens.

Threats to Validity

The validity of a study rests on the accuracy of the relationships between the dependent and independent variables. Therefore, there were some key issues that could threaten the validity of this study. Nongeneralizability of the study could threaten its external validity. For example, this study focused on women in three cities in Texas (Dallas, Houston, and San Antonio). Thus, the research outcome may not be applied to women in other cities. As this was a randomized, quasi-experimental research study, it was further possible that certain issues could reduce its internal validity. For example, existence of confound bias could render the whole study invalid.

The confounding variables in this study were hypovitaminosis D, inadequate metabolisms of vitamin D, abnormal Vitamin D gene Receptors or *single nucleotide polymorphisms* (SNPs), and lack of regular breast screenings. Existence of confound bias could lead to inability to draw conclusions in regard to whether a dependent variable influenced an independent variable to lead to a disease outcome. According to Armistead (2014) and Ohanuka (2017), it is not possible to completely eliminate problems emanating from a third variable. However, in this study, an attempt was made to minimize the confounding biases by controlling for the covariates. For example, individuals who could not have optimal exposure to sunlight were excluded from the study. In addition to this, individuals whose first-degree relations had been diagnosed with breast cancer were excluded.

In a breast cancer study, it is possible that *social desirability* bias may arise. This occurs in situations where an individual provides a "favorable image" response or a misguided response or gives wrong answers to questions when they feel uncomfortable with the situation. Furthermore, in situations where a survey is used in obtaining data from participants, it is possible that not all the questions would be answered accurately (Creswell, 2009). In this study, it might be possible that this situation arose, particularly as a survey was used in determining knowledge, exposure to sunlight, and frequency of breast examinations. To minimize inaccurate responses, efforts were made to phrase the questions carefully, and this was also done in order to avoid asking embarrassing questions. Furthermore, to reduce the effects of social desirability bias, efforts were made to review the data received from participants. Thus, extreme scores and outliers were checked for, and were adjusted accordingly.

Breast Cancer Preview

Breast cancer accounts for 22.9% of all female cancers and is the most common malignancy among women worldwide (Alharb et al., 2011; Ferlay et al., 2010). In the United States, breast cancer accounts for 26% of all cancers among women. It is also a major health problem among African American and Caucasian women (Susan G. Komen, 2017). According to the National Cancer Institute (2010), one in eight women will be diagnosed with breast cancer in their lifetime. In the United States, breast cancer is not only the most commonly diagnosed malignant disease among women but also the second leading cause of cancer-related deaths among women (American Cancer Society, 2015). Furthermore, it has been estimated that in 2017 there would be about 252,710 new cases of invasive breast cancer and 63,410 new cases of noninvasive (in situ) breast cancer diagnoses in women in the United States. It was further estimated that about 40,610 women in the United States would die from breast cancer in 2017 (National Breast Cancer Foundation, 2016).

The exact causes of breast cancer are not known; thus, only the risk factors are usually discussed. Furthermore, extrapolations from previous researches revealed that many women, especially African American women, have been consistently unaware of the risk factors associated with breast cancer. Therefore, the risk factors need to be discussed. One of the significant risk factors associated with breast cancer is Vitamin D Receptor gene polymorphism. Nevertheless, adequate intake of Vitamin D and exposure to ambient sunlight could effectively reduce breast cancer prevalence among women.

The Risk Factors for Breast Cancer

Although the exact causes of breast cancer are not known, there are a number of risk factors associated with the disease. The following are some of the risk factors.

Genetics. Breast cancer can develop through a number of mutations, in either the genes or in the breast cells. Thus, some inheritable genetic mutations may increase a person's chances of getting breast cancer. For example, individuals who are carriers of BRCA1 and BRCA2 genes have about 65–85% higher risks of developing breast cancer, whereas the average population without that gene has about a 12% chance of developing the disease.

Telomerase. This is an enzyme that has reverse transcriptase. Thus, it has RNA-dependent DNA polymerase activity. This enzyme is expressed in both stem cells and cancer cells. Cancer cells are immortal. They elude apoptosis. Therefore, they continue to divide indefinitely, without aging; and their telomeres never shorten.

Gender. According to the National Cancer Institute (2015), women are 100 times more likely to be diagnosed with breast cancer than men.

Age. A woman's chance of affliction with breast cancer increases as she advances in age. Statistically, each year, about 17% of women 40 years of age and 70% of women 50 years of age or older are diagnosed with breast cancer (National Cancer Institute, 2007).

Ethnicity (or race). Generally, Caucasian women are more predisposed to breast cancer than African American women (National Cancer Institute, 2007). However, at younger ages (between 40 to 50, African American women have a higher incidence of breast cancer than Caucasian women. Also, African American women are more likely to die from breast cancer than any other ethnic group (American Cancer Society, 2016).

Family history. A person is at high risk for breast cancer if her first-degree relative (i.e., mother, daughter, or sister) has been diagnosed with breast cancer.

Personal history of breast cancer. A person who had previously been diagnosed with breast cancer has a higher risk of breast cancer recurrence.

Sedentary lifestyle. Women who do not exercise are at higher risk for breast cancer than those who do. Moderate exercise of 3 or more hours a week may decrease a woman's breast cancer risk by more than 30% (Wood, 2008).

Breastfeeding history. Women who never breastfed are at higher risk for breast cancer than the general population.

Menstrual history. Early menarche (i.e., women whose menstrual flow started at an early age or before age 12), and late menopause (i.e., women who reached menopause after age 55), are more at risk for developing breast cancer.

Environment. Poor diet (fried foods, foods high in saturated fat, no fruits and vegetables), being overweight or obese, and exposure to radiation can increase a woman's risk for breast cancer.

Inverted nipple. Inverted nipple or benign breast mutations can increase the risk for breast cancer.

Pregnancy history. Nulliparity or not bearing children, late pregnancy (i.e., women whose first pregnancy occurred at more than 35 years of age) have higher chances of developing breast cancer than the general population.

Hormone replacement therapy. Therapies involving estrogen and progesterone can increase the risk for breast cancer.

Alcoholism. Heavy alcohol consumption heightens breast cancer risks. The risk factors for breast cancer are summarized in Figure 7.

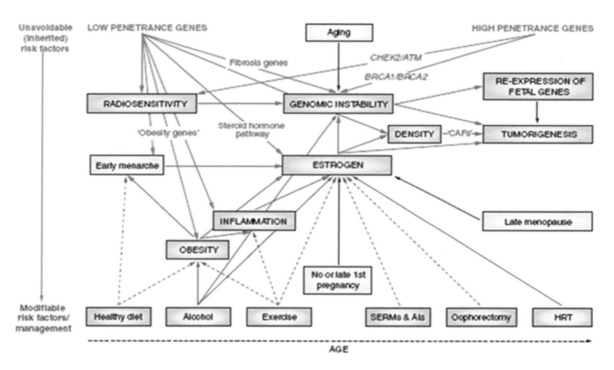

*Figure 7.*Summary of risk factors for breast cancer. Adapted *from Images for Health Belief Model,* by Jones & Bartlett Learning (2016). (www.jblearning.com/samples/0763743836/)

The Role of Mammograms and Breast Self-Exams

According to the National Cancer Institute (2017) and the Center for Disease Control and Prevention (2014), death rates among African American women due to breast cancer continue to rank highest in the United States when compared to other races. Women of all ages who perform regular breast self-examinations, and women from 40 years of age and above who perform regular clinical breast examinations (or mammograms), might have 90% chances of being cured from breast cancer due to early detection. In the Southern United States, 380 women ≥30 years of age were assessed for their use of BSE and mammograms. It was found that only 27% of the women performed BSE, and only 6.8% of women used mammograms to screen for breast cancer. For this reason, the current study used SurveyMonkey approach to reach a broad spectrum of participants in order to assess subjects' levels of awareness and/or knowledge concerning the disease, and inculcate in them a sense of urgency and intentions to perform regular breast self-exams and mammograms in an effort to minimize breast cancer exacerbation.

Mammograms and breast self-exams (BSE) are important screenings that can help in early detection of breast cancer. While BSE should be performed by women of all ages, the American Cancer Society (2013) recommends that women ≥40 years of age should submit to yearly clinical mammographic screenings. Regular mammograms and early cancer detection make a difference in staging breast cancer. Undoubtedly, these can save lives. African American women consistently have lower rates of mammographic screenings than Caucasian women. Lack of BSE and low rates of mammograms are part of the reasons African American women have a larger incidence of deaths from breast cancer than Caucasian women.

However, due to increased awareness of the risk factors, the rate of African American women submitting to mammograms has increased from 49% to 67%. Even though detection is more difficult in younger women and in women with dense breasts, mammograms are often helpful in detecting breast cancer before the manifestation of any symptoms (American Cancer Society, 2015). For this reason, mammograms play a pivotal role in saving lives.

African American women have a low rate of using mammographic screening due to several factors. One is lack of knowledge. The other factors include spiritual beliefs—for example, the faith that God will heal them and will not let any evil befall them. Thus, this imaginary fountain of hope for the hopeless maximizes their faith and expectations that they will be healed through miracles. It is therefore not uncommon that a woman of African descent would rather go to a pastor (than to go see a medical doctor), and request for prayers, incantations or conjurations for cure of a deadly disease, which simple surgery could have remedied at an early stage, when there had been no nodal formation or distant spread. Such patient believes that the pastor's supplications and intercessions would bring GOD's favor to her, and He will see her through the situation.

Similarly, some believe that breast cancer is daemonic and that the pastor, through "powerful spiritual means", could cast out the "daemonic spirit of cancer". Therefore, she would adhere to the pastor's suggested regimen to use traditional medicine to drive the "Daemon" out and bring her cure. Meanwhile, the cancer would keep spreading. Under normal circumstances, she could have had a good chance for a cure as well as a good chance of preserving her breasts had she not opted out of medical treatment in want of traditional medicine.

In essence, the African American woman may not go for breast cancer screenings or attend to breast cancer treatment regimens because she believes that as long as she does her daily prayers and is in good atonement with the Supreme Deity that God will miraculously heal her breast cancer. Another similar reason why African American women fall behind in breast cancer screening may be religious syncretism, or the cultural belief that their ancestors or some deities are watching over them and will prevent catastrophic illnesses from weighing them down. Thus, they believe, God cannot give a person a burden s/he cannot handle.

Fatalism, or the belief that breast cancer is beyond human control, is another factor that may delay an African American woman from going for breast cancer screenings or seeking treatment. Lack of medical insurance coverage is yet another reason why black women delay treatment, especially if the person cannot afford paying for the medical treatments.

Furthermore, perceived substandard medical treatments African Americans receive in hospitals compared to their Caucasian American counterparts could be another factor preventing this ethnic group from going for required breast cancer screenings and treatment programs. Disparities in mammographic screenings among African American women can also be attributed to such socioeconomic factors as poor income (or poverty), lack of education or awareness about the disease, and the demographic or geographic areas where they live.

Research has also shown that, when compared to Caucasian women, African American women do not follow the U.S. Preventive Services Task Force (USPSTF) mammography screening guideline, which recommends annual screenings for women ≥40 years of age (Jones et al., 2007; Mangum, 2016; USPSTF, 2017). This, among other factors, could lead to late-stage breast cancer and disproportionate death rates among African American women as compared to Caucasian American women.

Assessment of Vitamin D Intake

Questionnaires have been an effective method of identifying Vitamin D deficiency in research participants. For example, in a study conducted by Bolek-Berquist et al. (2009), a questionnaire was administered to a convenient sample of female adults in Madison, Wisconsin. Each participant's serum Vitamin D level was measured using a chemiluminescent assay. Serum Vitamin D level of <16 ng/ml. was defined as deficient. Serum concentration levels ranging from 50 nmol/L to 72 nmol/L were defined as significantly insufficient; and a serum concentration level greater than 72 nmol/L was deemed physiologically sufficient (Goodwin, Ennis, Pritchard, Koo, & Hood, 2009). According to Holick (2007), the ideal serum concentration level of Vitamin

D should not be below 75 nmol/L but should be between 75 nmol/L and 150 nmol/L. The idea is to avoid hypovitaminosis D (low serum vitamin D), which may lead to breast cancer; and also to prevent hypervitaminosis D (or excessive level of vitamin D), which can lead to Vitamin D toxicity—a potentially harmful effect.

A person's daily intake of Vitamin D should be between 800 and 1000 IU (International Units). This would help maintain adequate levels of Vitamin D in serum. This could also help promote physiologic health effects and prevent breast pathogenesis. In this research, there were two ways through which levels of Vitamin D intake were assessed. One was through hospital records, and the other was by relying on the information supplied by the participants.

Where hospital records were not available, participants' responses regarding their daily sunlight exposure were relied on. Thus, to ascertain the average of a participant's daily Vitamin D intake, her number of hours of exposure per week, was added to the dosage amount of any Vitamin D supplements she took. The figure was then divided by 7 (days of the week). Through the survey, individuals who were photophobic or photosensitive and/or those who could not maintain the recommended level of Vitamin D intake were excluded. The questions used in the survey to assess participants' knowledge for breast cancer can be seen in Appendix B.

The Role of Vitamin D Receptor gene Polymorphisms in Cancer Risk

The roles Vitamin D Receptor (VDR) gene polymorphisms play in various types of cancers (including cancers of the breast, prostate, ovary, colon, skin, bladder, and kidney), have been a subject of great inquiry among epidemiologists. To this end, previous researchers have analyzed the associations between Vitamin D Receptor gene polymorphisms FokI, BsmI, TaqI, and ApaI and breast cancer risks among African American and Caucasian women. However, the outcomes of the analyses have been inconclusive.

The Role of Vitamin D & Sunlight Exposure in Breast Cancer Prevention

There is growing evidence that Vitamin D and sunlight exposure play a protective role against breast cancer. It is therefore assumed that the integral role of Vitamin D is to prevent breast cancer and abnormal mitotic cell divisions, and thus maintain a holistic health effect in the human person. In a case-control analysis involving 91 breast cancer patients, it was revealed that 87% of the patients had triple negative breast cancer as a result of low serum vitamin D, and the remaining 13% of the patients presented with other subtypes of breast cancer (Azizi et al., 2009).

Consistent with that finding, another study conducted on some volunteers also revealed that individuals with 90 nmol/L of Vitamin D (25D3) in their serums were in normal physiological statuses, while patients with breast cancer had as low as 50 nmol/L level of Vitamin D in their serums (Rainville, Khan, & Tisman, 2009). Furthermore, in a case-control study involving more than 8,200 breast cancer women (4,100 cases and 4,100 controls), it was found that daily intake of 400 IU of supplemental Vitamin D was associated with a decrease in breast cancer risk (Anderson et al., 2010).

Also, in a longitudinal study involving more than 67,000 women, Engel et al. (2011) reported that adequate intake of supplemental vitamin D, along with sunlight exposure, was statistically significant in reducing breast cancer risk. Additionally, a meta-analysis was conducted on 21 studies in which Vitamin D blood levels were evaluated among the participants. The results indicated that women with the highest level of serum Vitamin D had a 45% decrease in breast cancer risk. On the other hand, low serum levels of Vitamin D have been implicated as a breast cancer risk.

On the contrary, some other researchers found no evidence of vitamin D involvement in breast cancer risk-reduction. For example, Kuper and Associates (2009) found no association between Vitamin D intake and breast cancer risk-reduction. Similarly, a meta-analysis that combined results of six studies reported that there was no association between Vitamin D (either from sunlight exposure or diet) and breast cancer risk. Equally, a longitudinal study involving more than 41,000 women found no link between Vitamin D intake and reduction in breast cancer risk (Chlebowski et al. 2008).

Nonetheless, amidst numerous contradictory reports concerning the role of Vitamin D in breast cancer prevention, evidence abounds supporting that Vitamin D promotes human health. However, the purpose of this study was not to place a judgment call on either side of the two spectra of claims, but rather to assess the involvement of Vitamin D and Vitamin D Receptor gene polymorphisms in breast cancer causation among the subject population. It was therefore the purpose of this study to assess how knowledge and awareness of the disease process influence decisions of women for behavior change toward reducing the prevalence of breast cancer. The study was theoretically guided by Roy's Adaptation Model (RAM).

Roy's Adaptation Model (RAM)

I chose Roy's Adaptation Model as the theoretical framework for this study because it has the five constructs of interest in this research:

- The health of the individual,
- The person (and her motivation, behaviors, beliefs, and attitudes),
- The health care personnel (nurse, physician) and readiness to educate and treat the person,
- The adaptation (willingness of the breast cancer patient to adapt and make changes— resilience, self-efficacy, and response efficacy), and
- The environment (modifiable factors affecting breast cancer—mammograms, exposure to sunlight, dietary supplements, and the like).

RAM views an individual person in a holistic way. The core concept of RAM is to help the person adapt. For this to happen, the healthcare system and its personnel must assume that a person is an open system capable of responding to stimuli from the internal and external aspects of the person (Roy & Andrews, 1999).

In this research, environment is seen as stimuli, which include contextual, behavioral, focal, and residual. Contextual stimuli include variables such as what the person eats (eating/drinking habits) and other causative factors, such as what the person is exposed to in the environment she comes in contact with. Focal stimuli represent immediate, apparent, and foreseeable causes of the problem or danger; this may include immediate and long-term effects of a person's lifestyle. Residual stimuli are issues relating to patients' past experiences with illnesses and how the experiences impact the patients' current condition. These stimuli—contextual, focal, and residual—were analyzed in this research in an effort to understand how best to reduce breast cancer incidence rates among the subject population.

Coping mechanisms during adverse situations or illness are physiological in nature and can be regulated or manipulated through *regulator* and *cognator* activities. These may range from physiological attributes to physical attributes to psychological or social attributes. The healthcare professional's role while caring for the patients involves manipulating the stimuli that come from the environment so that they fall within the patient's field of positive coping, resulting in adaptation. Adaptation should therefore be considered as an effective response to a stimulus, while a negative response should be considered as an ineffective approach to a stimulus involving patient disease-prevention methodology. According to Naga et al. (2014), adaptation can take place in four modes—one physiological mode and three psychosocial modes, which include (a) self-concept, awareness, or knowledge; (b) role function, participation in healthcare program, taking initiative or response efficacy; and (c) interdependence). The four modes are an interrelated concept.

Finally, I chose RAM because it is one of the theoretical frameworks most frequently used in researches that educate patients in healthcare settings and practices. Therefore, RAM was the right theoretical framework to guide this study in answering the research questions and testing the hypotheses.

Importance of Knowledge in Reducing Breast Cancer Risk

Under normal circumstances, it is reasonable to believe that people would likely adapt to a new health behavior if there were perceived benefits than when there were perceived barriers or obstacles. In this case, the perceived benefit was applying an acquired knowledge toward reduction of breast cancer risks.

On this axiom, Alharbi, Alshammar, Almutairi, Makboul, and El-Shazly (2011) conducted a study among Kuwaiti female schoolteachers assessing their knowledge, awareness, behaviors, and practices concerning breast cancer risk-reduction. As shown in Figure 8 below, 384 women were contacted in the initial telephone interview. Only 290 of the women agreed to participate in the breast cancer educational program. The results of the study revealed that 67.5% of the participants had knowledge about breast cancer. The researchers indicated that 98.2% of the sources of breast cancer information were from health professionals and health workers, while about 83.5% of the knowledge and awareness about the disease came from friends and neighbors. Furthermore, about 76.0% of the information came from TV and radio, and 60.2% came from printed materials.

Ejike R. Egwuekwe

Therefore, printed materials, banners, radio/TV shows, professional bodies, and church bulletins became the principal channel through which the outcome of my research was disseminated. Among the participants in this research, about 18.5% reported a positive family history of breast cancer, 49.9% did not know how to perform breast self-exams, and 29.0% knew about the procedure but never practiced it. Also, 81.9% never had any breast examination by healthcare professionals, and 85.7% did not know anything about mammograms. This research further revealed an insufficient knowledge among these female participants in respect to breast cancer. It further exemplified the negative influence of low knowledge on the practice of using mammograms and breast self-exams as necessary measures for early breast cancer detection.

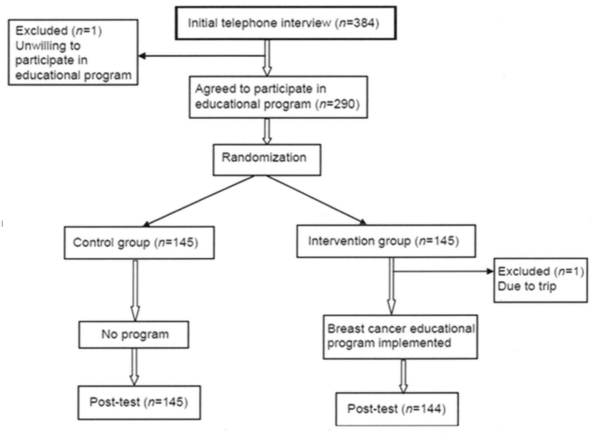

Figure 8. Participants in a breast cancer educational program. From "Knowledge, Awareness, and Practices Concerning Breast Cancer among Kuwaiti Female School Teachers," by Alharbi et al., 2012, *Alexandria Journal of Medicine*, 48, pp. 75–82.

Response Efficacy

Response efficacy is a motivational belief system. It can help a person to evaluate his or her response to a recommended action and appreciate or refute its effectiveness.

Perloff (2013) indicated that direct persuasion and indirect persuasion could be used in getting autism patients to enroll in treatment programs. I applied this concept in effectively getting breast cancer patients to enroll in therapies. In like manner, breast cancer awareness programs, education and interpersonal communication forums were effectively utilized, as they played important roles in changing patient's attitudes toward treatment programs.

According to Champion (1999), response efficacy occurs through a construct of perceived benefits. This can occur when a woman perceives the benefits of mammographic screening and believes that obtaining a mammogram can help her find breast lumps early. Sometimes, however, a woman may believe that mammography might help others detect breast cancer early, but not necessarily believe it would do so for herself. This is a sense of perceived hopelessness and helplessness. This can lead to delay in seeking treatment. Such delay can be fatal.

Lack of belief that mammographic screenings can be helpful in early detection of breast cancer might be due to fatalism. It might also be due to personal and cultural beliefs. Fatalism could in turn be tied to perceptions of hopelessness, helplessness, worthlessness, meaninglessness, powerlessness, and social despair. A person trapped in such a belief system may believe that cancer is beyond his or her personal control. Thus, they believe that nothing can be done to change such a negative situation as breast cancer.

Nevertheless, response efficacy could motivate individuals to assess the benefits of breast cancer screening and analyze their behaviors toward breast self-examination. This concept has been successfully applied toward mammography. For example, perceived benefits for mammograms could be a determining factor as to whether a woman enrolled in a program or not. On this premise, perceived benefits could be defined as an inducement that motivates a person to positively respond to cancer treatment programs. Perceived benefits, or the lack thereof, make a difference in regard to whether a woman decides to go for a mammogram, actually goes, and continues to go and adhere to the mammographic process.

A significant motivator or benefit that differentiated between those women who thought about it and those who actually performed a mammogram could be the value attributed to finding lumps early. It could also be due to a desire to decrease chances of dying from breast cancer. Furthermore, the motivator could be perceived benefits in using mammography as a helpful tool in finding lumps before they can be felt. However, in a study among a group of low-income African American women, perceptions of these benefits were lower, whereas the perceptions were higher among Caucasian American women. Figure 9 shows women's attitudes toward having a mammogram.

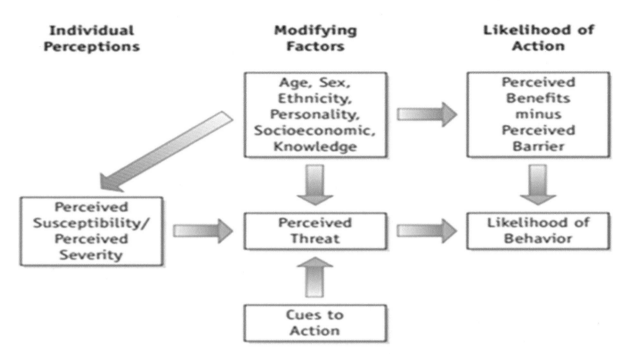

Figure 9. Perceptions and motivations for breast cancer screenings. Adapted from *The Health Belief Model* (pp. 39–62), K. Glanz, F. M. Lewis,& B. K. Rimer, 2015, San Francisco, CA: Jossey-Bass.

Perceived Barriers to Mammograms

Research has shown that there are various barriers that prevent some women from going for breast cancer screenings until it is too late. For example, in a research conducted among 9,000 women at the Siteman Cancer Center Mammography Outreach Registry in Missouri, 40% of the women stated that cost of mammograms was a major hindrance to them (Fayanju, Kraenzle, Drake, Oka, & Goodman, 2014). Additionally, 13% of the women claimed that mammogram-related pain was a significant barrier to them, while another 13% indicated that they were afraid of receiving bad news. Also, some women might have been afraid that their husbands, boyfriends, or significant others would leave them in the event of a positive breast cancer diagnosis.

Among African women, breast cancer is usually diagnosed in late stages—in most cases because of personal beliefs, limited resources, or low socioeconomic status. For example, in a cross-sectional, randomized study conducted among 612 Egyptian women, it was found that 81.8% of the women would not go for checkups unless they became ill. Another 77% revealed their unwillingness to have a mammogram unless it was recommended by their doctor (Mamdouh et al., 2014).Furthermore, 71.4% of the women indicated that they were shy and would not go for mammograms due to "lack of privacy." Another 69.2% of the women believed that medical checkups were not necessary and not worth their time, and 64.6% said they would not go for breast cancer screenings because of the cost of services.

As shown in Figure 10, the reasons why some women feel reluctant to go for breast cancer screening include cultural and religious influences, social injustices, low socioeconomic status, and poverty. Also, women with lower education, women from lower income categories, unemployed women, and women who have poor knowledge of the risks of breast cancer are likely to be indifferent to mammographic procedures. Further, women who have no family history of breast cancer are more likely to be indifferent, nonchalant, or apathetic toward breast cancer screenings compared with their counterparts or those with personal or familial histories of the disease.

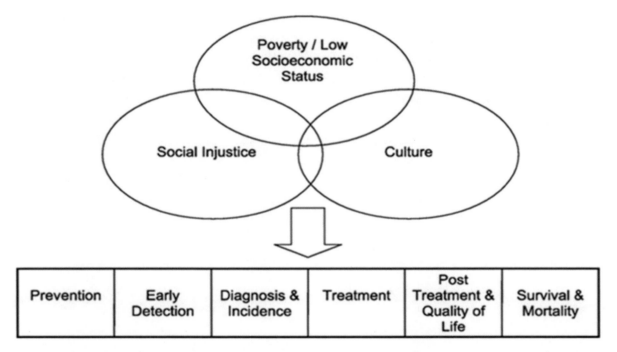

Figure 10. Three interrelated factors preventing most African American women from going for breast cancer screening. Adapted *from Images for Health Belief Model,* by Jones & Bartlett Learning (2016). (www.jblearning.com/samples/0763743836/)

Perceived Benefits of Breast Cancer Screenings

Domenighetti et al. (2003) conducted a research in four countries: the United States, the United Kingdom, Italy, and Switzerland. The research involved 5,964 women aged 15 and older. The research found that 68% of Caucasian women believed that screening could help prevent or reduce the risk of contracting breast cancer. In another study conducted among 414 Iranian women aged 40 to 73 years, Allahverdipour, Asghari-Jafarabadi, and Emami (2011) found that 29% of the women performed at least one mammogram due to the perceived benefits of screening. This was particularly true if the women were older, or if they had personal/familial histories of breast cancer, or if they had a history of any breast disease. Having health insurance coverage and living in an urban area where healthcare is available are some other factors that could promote involvement in mammograms.

Furthermore, it is possible that the desire for regular mammographic screenings correlates with differences in age, residence areas, educational levels, hormone replacement therapy status, and history of breast cancer. For example, in this research, women in the older age groups, with a higher educational level, in receipt of hormone replacement therapy, and with a personal history of breast cancer believed it was beneficial to engage in breast cancer screening. This group of women would have significantly higher odds ratios for regular mammograms. This could reduce their risks for breast cancer and probably save their lives.

One of the barriers that prevented African American women from engaging in regular mammographic screening was that they were less adequately informed about breast cancer screening than were Caucasian women. Inadequate access to health information could lead to inaction. This could also encourage apathy and disinterest among this ethnic group in respect to mammograms. Figure 11 reveals an array of barriers that could hinder women from engaging in breast cancer screenings. These may include cultural, religious, or personal beliefs; fear of being diagnosed; socioeconomic reasons; and barriers due to the health system itself. In some cases, the barriers might originate from lack of knowledge or awareness. Whatever the case may be, the barriers need to be identified and addressed so that the target population would be encouraged to adopt behavioral change necessary to save their lives. The best way to disseminate breast cancer information to reach the African American women is through churches, billboards, and community-based forums. On the other hand, breast cancer research outcome can be disseminated through many channels including magazines, books, newspaper articles, television shows, to reach Caucasian women.

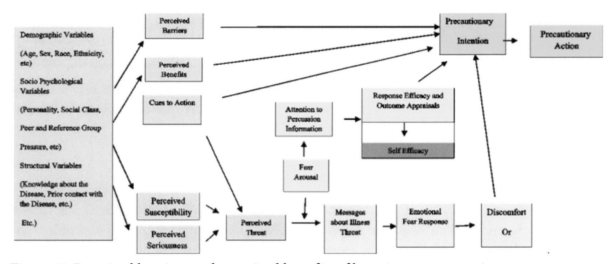

Figure 11. Perceived barriers and perceived benefits of breast cancer screenings. Adapted *from Images and Graphs for Health Belief Model,* by Jones & Bartlett Learning, 2016. (www.Jblearning.com/samples/076373836/chapter%204.pdf)

Summary

Breast cancer is a dreadful disease of unknown etiology. It accounts for 22.9% of all female cancers around the world and 26% of all cancers among women in the United States. In the United States, 1 in 8 women will be diagnosed with breast cancer in their lifetime (National Cancer Institute, 2010). It was also estimated that more than 40,610 women in the United States would die from breast cancer in 2017 (National Breast Foundation, 2016). Although the statistics changes from year to year, it has always been on the increase. Research should focus on how to bring down the morbidity and mortality rates. This was the central element of my research.

Previous researchers have usually discussed only the risk factors of breast cancer (Engel et al., 2011). Even so, it has not been discussed at the level of the individual. This has left a gap in literature worthy of investigation. The gap became the void that this research sought to fill. For example, Mohr et al. (2008) and the National Cancer Foundation (2015) indicated that many African American women are unaware of the risk factors associated with breast cancer. On that axiom, this research adopted various means to raise awareness of the subject population in respect to breast cancer risk factors. One of the significant risk factors associated with breast cancer in African American and Caucasian women is Vitamin D Receptor gene polymorphism. Exposure to sunlight and/or supplementary Vitamin D could be used to reduce this risk.

This chapter discussed the literature search strategy, the risk factors for breast cancer, and the roles of mammograms and breast self-exam in early cancer detection. This chapter also discussed the associations of Vitamin D and Vitamin D Receptor gene polymorphisms in breast cancer risks and the subjects' levels of application of knowledge, behaviors, and attitudes in the disease management process. As shown on Figure 11 above, there is no doubt that an array of barriers could potentially prevent some women from engaging in breast cancer screenings. The barriers might include cultural, religious, or personal beliefs, fear of being diagnosed, socioeconomic reasons, and other barriers associated with the health system itself. In some cases, the barriers originate from lack of knowledge or awareness. Whatever the case might be, the barriers need to be identified and addressed. Identifying and addressing the problems could encourage the target population to adopt behavioral change necessary to save their lives.

However, knowledge alone cannot change behavior. Cultural attributes and beliefs could influence a person's decisions to change a given behavior in respect to health situations, including mammograms and response to breast cancer treatments. Thus, for individuals to respond effectively to mammographic screenings, it is imperative to focus on cultural traditions when educating patients about the importance and methods of breast self-exams and mammographic screenings. Culture, therefore, can be integrated the milieu of treatment regimens.

Addressing the barriers by increasing women's awareness of breast cancer, addressing the misconceptions women have regarding breast examinations, and educating the subjects on the importance of Vitamin D in breast cancer risk reduction can help policy makers in designing breast cancer treatment programs culturally suitable for respective ethnic groups. Furthermore, the individual would have to take an active part in behaviors to change the outcome of a perceived dreadful illness. Because RAM contains the five intrinsic elements guiding health adaptations, it was chosen as the theoretical concept that guided this study. Chapter 3 discusses the research design, the rationale for adopting the research design, and the methodology used in this study. Chapter 3 also discusses the sample size, the research procedure, the demographics, and the ethical considerations in this research.

Chapter 3: Research Method

Introduction

The objective of this quantitative, quasi-experimental study was to assess the knowledge/awareness of the link between VDR gene polymorphisms and the risks of breast cancer among women in Texas, in the Southern United States. SurveyMonkey method was used to distribute survey questionnaires to the participants. The data obtained were used to assess participants' levels of awareness, knowledge, and behaviors in respect to breast cancer and breast cancer risk-reduction practices.

The RAM theory guided this study. The method of inquiry was approached by looking at the subjects' levels of education and awareness in respect to the disease process. Also, I explored the participants' rates of exposure to sunlight and/or their intake of supplemental vitamin D. The participants' readiness to respond to breast cancer screening and their attitude toward breast cancer risk reduction were also assessed. In this chapter, the research design, sample size, experimental procedure, instrument administration, and ethical considerations are discussed.

Research Design and Rationale

This was a quantitative, quasi-experimental study, whose subjects were served questionnaires through SurveyMonkey approach. The survey was randomized, and the age of interest ranged from 20 to 70. The participants were selected from three major cities in the state of Texas. The cities of interest were Houston, San Antonio, and Dallas.

I chose a randomized approach because each of the cities of interest is large. Therefore, randomization was the only reasonable approach to draw participants and minimize selection bias. Further, these three cities in Texas were chosen to ensure that the areas of coverage were ones with adequate amount of sunlight. It was necessary to ensure that the participants had equal chances of exposure to sunlight. Anyone whose culture or religion or job or medical condition did not permit them to have direct exposure to sunlight, or anyone who had sunlight sensitivity or photophobia, was excluded unless she had equal access to supplemental or dietary vitamin D. The survey material was presented in eighth-grade English. Therefore, it was presumed that each participant was able to read at an eighth-grade level. Individuals who could not read or write at the eighth-grade level were excluded from the study.

The rationales for selecting the participants through SurveyMonkey method were (a) to make sure the three big cities of interest were sufficiently covered and (b) to make sure that sufficient representative samples were obtained. For example, it is the policy of SurveyMonkey to supply more subjects in the event additional participants are required. Because the three cities (Dallas, Houston, and San Antonio) are several hundreds of miles apart, using any other means to recruit participants would not have been feasible.

Participants, Sample Size, and Rationale

Participants in this research were African American and Caucasian American women between the ages of 20 and 70. As can be seen in Table 1, breast cancer can start in a woman as early as 20 years of age.

Table 1

Absolute Risk of Breast Cancer in U. S. Women by Age

If current age is:	Absolute risk of developing breast cancer in the next 10 years is:
20	1 in 1,760 (0.06%)
30	1 in 229 (0.4%)
40	1 in 69 (1.4%)
50	1 in 42 (2.4%)
60	1 in 29 (3.4%)
70	1 in 27 (3.7%)

Note: The older a woman gets, the higher her absolute risk of getting breast cancer. Adapted from "Absolute Risk of Breast Cancer in U. S. Women," by Susan G. Komen, 2017. (http://ww5.kome.org/KomenPerspectives/Breast-cancer-statistics-made-easy.html).

According to the American Cancer Society (2013), the aggressive and more deadly species of breast cancer can occur among the African American population at an early age of 20 years, but not among the Caucasian American women. The reason is yet to be defined.

The sample size used in this study was drawn from three major cities in Texas–Houston, San Antonio, and Dallas. Because of the size of these three big cities, SurveyMonkey approach was the only practicable approach through which the participants could be reached. SurveyMonkey could offer a substantial assistance in recruiting survey participants, as its services were available 24 hours a day, 7 days a week, all year round. One important reason for choosing participants from these cities was to ensure that the participants were of equal or similar socioeconomic statuses, living in the same time zone with similar geographic conditions, and exposed to similar degrees of sources of vitamin D, either through direct sunlight or dietary supplementation.

Women who were allergic to dietary or supplemental vitamin D, or women who had photophobia or sunlight sensitivity, or women who could not be exposed to the direct sunlight for any reasons, including for medical or religious reasons, were excluded. Women who could not read or write or understand the materials written in simple English were excluded. This was to make sure that each participant understood basic instructions in the survey material. These exclusions were made so as to minimize threats to the validity of the study.

Additionally, women with previous breast cancer diagnoses were excluded. Similarly, women who had suffered any number of diseases suggesting possible mutations in the p53, BRCA1, and BRCA2 genes were excluded from the study. Mutations in the p53 and BRCA genes are potential breast cancer risks. Therefore, excluding these women would reduce biases that could affect the validity of the study.

In using the SurveyMonkey method, effort was made to contact the participants through five steps. Initial letters were sent out informing recipients that they would be receiving an e-mail to participate in an Internet survey. This was followed by e-mails indicating the link where the survey was to be taken. Next, postcards were sent out thanking the participants. Subsequently, e-mails were resent to all nonrespondents. In all interactions and communications with participant, effort was made to maintain ethical standards.

Using SurveyMonkey method was beneficial because it helped achieve a high response rate. For example, this approach used questionnaires that were simple and easy to understand by the respondents. Also, an e-mail address and stamped return envelopes were sent to potential participants, making it easier for respondents to return survey materials either by e-mail or by post, whichever way they chose. The stamped envelopes, phone calls, postcards, and hand-written reminders were steps taken to add a personal touch to the survey.

Additionally, SurveyMonkey method was used in distributing breast cancer self-awareness information to the respondents, because I wished to educate individuals on the importance of being screened, and using this method enabled me to reach a vast majority of people. I also included information about the risks of late-stage breast cancer and information on breast cancer symptoms. Information about the importance of making healthy lifestyle choices, the need to exercise regularly and to avoid a sedentary lifestyle was also included.

The purpose of the research was explained to the participants. The participants were not offered any sort of compensation, remuneration, rewards, incentives, or benefits to participate in the study. However, they were advised that they could receive a copy of the research outcome if they desired. The participants were also informed that they had the right to withdraw their consent at any time, either before or during the research process, without any question. Their consents were, therefore, voluntary.

Procedures

Survey Instrument Administration

The survey instrument was administered to 250 female participants. The sampling frame included individuals who volunteered, individuals from households and institutions that received survey materials, and individuals willing to participate. There were 125 breast cancer cases and 125 controls who were recruited for the study. In the case category, 75 women were premenopausal, and 75 were postmenopausal. Similarly, in the control category, 75 women were premenopausal and 75 women were postmenopausal. The numbers were evenly distributed in both control and cases categories. This arrangement met a reasonable and realistic objective for the study. The survey materials that included informed consent forms were mailed out to each participant for completion.

Instrumentation and Materials

In the questionnaires, I focused on the participants' demographic characteristics, including, age, level of education, gender, ethnicity, and personal/family histories of breast cancer. The survey instrument also included questions on dependent variables assessing the participants' knowledge about breast cancer and breast cancer risk factors (including whether they knew that VDR gene polymorphisms could increase their susceptibility to breast cancer and whether they knew that increased accessibility to Vitamin D could reduce their susceptibility to breast cancer). Other dependent variables were participants' level of knowledge about breast self-examinations (BSEs) and their periodic use of mammograms. Other areas addressed by the questionnaire included assessment of participants' Vitamin D intake and their willingness to enroll in breast cancer risk-reduction programs.

Assessment of Breast Cancer Knowledge

Responses to educational level were assessed along with breast cancer knowledge. This helped in discriminating between the two variables (educational variable and breast cancer knowledge) to ensure that the two variables did not influence each other or that one was not attributable to the other. The questionnaire material was presented in simple English to ensure that respondents understood the information presented to them. Also, the questionnaire included a section where I assessed the participants' levels of resilience and response efficacy. In this part of the questionnaire, I assessed whether knowledge of, and worries about, breast cancer were likely to increase participants' willingness to respond to treatment programs.

All questions administered to the participants, except those that inquired about risk factors and symptoms of breast cancer, had three possible answer options (*yes, no,* and *not sure*). I used this approach to reveal the extent of lack of awareness and level of knowledge regarding breast cancer and treatment program involvement. The responses for each research question carried a score. The standards of questions in the questionnaire were adopted from the Canadian Cancer Society and the National Cancer Institute, USA. Table 2 gives a summary of grading criteria showing the level of knowledge in respect to breast cancer and early detection methods among women.

Table 2

Women's Level of Knowledge About Breast Cancer Early Detection

Serial number	Range of knowledge	Grading of knowledge
1	0-7	Very low knowledge
2	8-13	Low knowledge
3	14-18	Adequate knowledge
4	19-22	Excellent knowledge

Note: The more knowledgeable a woman is about breast cancer early detection, the more likely she would be to submit to regular mammogram. Adapted from "Developing a Research Instrument to Document Awareness, Knowledge, and Attitudes Regarding Breast Cancer and Early Detection Techniques for Pakistani Women: The Breast Cancer Inventory (BCI)," by A. A. Naqvi, F. Zehra, R. Ahmad, & N. Ahmad, 2016. (www.mdpi.com/2079-9721/4/4/37/pdf)

Assessment of Response Efficacy

For the purpose of this research, response efficacy can be defined as the extent to which an individual believes that participating in a recommended program can effectively diminish or alleviate a health threat. The survey administered to the respondents included questions regarding response efficacy and resilience. A sample of the questionnaire can be found in Appendix D. The method used was helpful in assessing the participants' drive, motivation, and likelihood to enlist in breast cancer risk-reduction programs.

To achieve the objective, a Likert Scale type of assessment was used. The participants were asked the following: On a scale of 1 to 5, how important is breast cancer screening to you and how important is Vitamin D intake to you? Similarly, they were asked (on a scale of 1 to 5) to indicate their resolve or determination to indulge in recommended programs. The Likert Scale type of assessment contained five levels of responses similar to the following: *strongly agree, agree, neither agree nor disagree, disagree, strongly disagree.*

Assessment for Resilience

According to Ristevska-Dimitrovska, Filov, Rajchanovska, Stefanovski, and Dejanova (2015), breast cancer patients who are resilient have better quality of life than those who are not resilient. The questionnaire, therefore, included questions that were used in assessing participants' knowledge/awareness in regard to VDR gene polymorphisms associated with breast cancer and their level of resilience and quality of life in relation to breast cancer. The questions that were used in assessing participants' level of knowledge/awareness of VDR polymorphisms can be found on Appendix C.

Research Design

The purpose of this study was to assess the associations between VDR gene polymorphisms and breast cancer risks among women in Texas, in the Southern United States. The objective was to understand the role played by VDR gene polymorphisms to increase breast cancer susceptibility among African American and Caucasian American women.

Research Questions and Hypotheses

The following research questions were addressed in this study:

1. Is there an association between VDR gene polymorphisms knowledge/awareness and decisions to reduce breast cancer risks?

$H_0 1$: There is no association between VDR gene polymorphisms knowledge/awareness and decisions to reduce breast cancer risks.

$H_a 1$: There is an association between VDR gene polymorphisms knowledge/awareness and decisions to reduce breast cancer risks.

2. Is there an association between knowledge of VDR gene polymorphisms and likelihood of mammogram screening?

$H_0 2$: There is no association between knowledge of VDR gene polymorphisms and likelihood of mammogram screening.

$H_a 2$: There is an association between knowledge of VDR gene polymorphisms and likelihood of mammogram screening.

Dependent Variables

Breast cancer was the dependent variable in this study. The following were the covariates: the level of knowledge about Vitamin D Receptor gene polymorphisms and it's disease process, education, awareness, and lifestyle such as cigarette smoking; exposure to sunlight for vitamin D; poor nutritional intake for supplementary vitamin D; and sedentary lifestyle and method of reducing breast cancer risk (such as breast self-exams and mammograms). In 2002, the USPSTF recommended that women from 40 years of age and older should submit to yearly mammograms. Based on this recommendation, the questionnaire used in this survey was designed to elicit information from the participants in relation to whether or not they had ever performed mammograms. The questions on the questionnaire in respect to mammogram screenings were easy and simple. For example, *yes* was used to indicate positive experience with mammographic examinations, and *no* was used to indicate never having had any such experience. The participants were also expected to indicate how many times (in number of years) they had performed mammograms and the age at which they first experienced one.

Independent Variables

The independent variables for this study were gender, age, socioeconomic status, early menarche, late menopause, and personal or family history of breast cancer. Resilience, response efficacy, perceived threats to personal health, perceived barriers to going for genetic tests for Vitamin D Receptor gene abnormalities (or polymorphisms), barriers to receiving treatments, and perceived benefits to mammograms were other independent variables explored in this study. These variables gave some insight into the disproportionate incidences in breast cancer morbidity and mortality rates among African American and Caucasian women. Reviewing these variables also was helpful in understanding why more Caucasian American women submit to mammographic screenings than African American women do. For example, reviewing these variables made it possible to understand that an average African American woman may not have health insurance or the financial resources to pay for breast cancer treatments, whereas her Caucasian American counterpart could afford the procedure.

Sample Selection

This study was based on a sample size of 250 African American and Caucasian women. The sample included women between 20 and 75 years of age and living in the urban areas of Dallas, Houston, and San Antonio. Using SurveyMonkey style was valuable in selecting the sample size. In addition to SurveyMonkey approach, another means for selecting sample size was through local churches, social centers, and senior center programs. As such, churches, community centers, and senior citizen center programs were good resources from which participants were recruited. These community social centers were instrumental resources for not only in distributing survey questionnaires but also in disseminating the research results. This is because these sources have many members that use their services. To achieve the goal of reaching a substantial number of people, pastors of the churches and directors of the senior service centers were used in delivering the message to members of these organizations.

Data Analysis

The survey data used in this quasi-experimental study were developed and disseminated to reach participants at least two or three months ahead of time, thereby giving them enough time to respond to the survey. Descriptive statistical analysis was performed using frequency, mean, and standard deviation. These were helpful in describing the basic features of the data used in the study. Inferential statistics, correlation and regression analyses were used in testing the hypotheses to answer the research questions. The allele frequency check was conducted with Hardy-Weinberg Equilibrium (equation): $p2 + 2pq + q2$. This is an equation that is normally used when calculating genetic allele frequencies. However, I found it prudent to use it in analyzing the presence of Vitamin D Receptor gene polymorphisms in breast cancer research.

For example, in this study, Hardy-Weinberg equilibrium was used in calculating the allele frequencies and in determining the homogeneity and heterogeneity of the alleles. In the equilibrium (or equation), p^2 represents the frequency of the homozygous genotype AA (i.e.,

Fok1 VDRFF). The q^2 represents the frequency for the homozygous genotype aa (i.e., Fok1 VDRff), and 2pq represents the frequency of the heterozygous genotype Aa (i.e., VDRFf). While there was no documentable evidence that previous researchers have looked at the heterogeneity as a potential source for cancer, such possibility exists. This finding should be researched and verified. The sum of the allele frequencies for all the alleles at the locus must add up to 1. Thus, $p + q = 1$, or 100%. Any departure from this norm would be anomalous. Therefore, this could be a potential source of cancer. In the meta-analysis study by Lu, Jing, and Zhang (2016), the heterogeneity was tested using the Cochrane Q statistic. The heterogeneity was considered not to be important if the P value was greater than 10($P > 0.10$).

Understanding the use and application of the Hardy-Weinberg equilibrium (equation) made it possible for me as a researcher to correct any entry mistakes and check for missing data and outliers. Thus, if a case was missing ≥50% or had up to ≥25% of missing data, the data was deleted from the data set, in accordance with the Stangor (2014) stipulation. Also, univariate outliers detected with the function were removed and replaced with the next lowest or highest value, also in accord with the Stangor stipulation. This stipulation is also in keeping with linear regression data analyses assumptions, compliance, and regulations, which require all data to be examined for potential outliers and to check for missing data (Rousseeuw & Leroy, 2003; Stangor, 2014).

The data analysis focused on the dependent variables, which included level of education, knowledge and awareness of breast cancer risk factors, and breast self-examinations. Other dependent variables were mammograms, lifestyle such as cigarette smoking, exposure to sunlight, poor nutritional intake, and sedentary lifestyle. Some other dependent variables were method of reducing breast cancer risk, resilience, and response efficacy. The independent variables included gender, age, early menarche, late menopause, and personal or family breast cancer history. The covariates were nulliparity, lack of breastfeeding, estrogen and/or progesterone replacement therapies, obesity, breast density, and alcoholism. Statistical tests were used in finding out whether the survey or the results of the experiment were significant. It helped in figuring out whether to reject the null hypotheses or accept the alternate hypotheses.

Ethical Considerations

Participants in this study were willing volunteers. They received no compensatory reward or benefit; neither in cash nor in kind. However, the participants were informed that they could receive a copy of the research outcome, should they choose to do so. Every participant had to sign an informed consent form, which was located on the first page of the questionnaire.

Furthermore, the participants were informed that they had the right to withdraw from the study at any point in time—before or during the study—without any consequences and without being asked their reasons for doing so. The researcher's contact information was provided on the cover page of the questionnaire, making it possible for the respondents to ask any questions at any time. Also, the contact information of the University Institutional Review Board (IRB) and the Research Chairperson or Supervisor was made available to the participants; these were also provided on the front page of the survey questionnaire. The respondents had to return the consent form together with the survey questionnaire in a timely fashion.

Ethical standards in research were strictly followed. For example, it is a standard operating procedure to subsequently dissociate the survey materials from the respondents' e-mail addresses, making it impossible to associate the responses with the respondents or the e-mails from whence they came. This was done. Furthermore, in order to maintain the highest standards of confidentiality and anonymity in respect to the participants, I, the researcher, also took measures to protect access to participants' identity. For example, Secure Sockets Layer (SSL) encryption was used to protect the data and the responses given by the participants. In addition to the foregoing, I made sure that the documents contained no identifying information with respect to the participants, thereby making it impossible for anyone to identify any of the participants by name or know how they responded to the survey questions. Also, I made sure that the Internet Protocol (IP) address tracking associated with the data collection was disabled, making it more difficult to trace or track any of the respondents through their original e-mail addresses.

Summary

The purpose of this study was to assess the associations of Vitamin D and Vitamin D Receptor gene polymorphisms as risk factors for breast cancer causation among women in Texas, in the Southern United States. The extent to which Vitamin D Receptor gene polymorphisms contribute to breast cancer exacerbation was ascertained through cancer registries, treatment centers, and hospital records. This was possible because Vitamin D (1,25-dihydroxy vitamin D3) has been recognized as a prophylaxis against breast cancer. It therefore has been adopted in breast cancer treatment regimens and therapies. Given that the actions of vitamin D3 are mediated through the Vitamin D Receptor (VDR), and because a number of polymorphisms in the VDR gene have been identified as breast cancer causative elements, I had to access cancer registries in search of data bearing evidence of such a claim. I used the data so obtained in measuring the variables.

To achieve the purpose of this research, the subjects' levels of knowledge and awareness about breast cancer risk factors, their behaviors toward the effects of Vitamin D Receptor gene polymorphisms in association with breast cancer risks, and their attitudes toward breast cancer risk reduction, were assessed.

The purpose of this chapter was to discuss the research methodology, the research design, and the method used in recruiting the participants. Sample size was also discussed, and so were survey instrumentation, data analysis, and ethical considerations. Chapter 4, coming up next, discusses the results of this research. The results are supported with tables and narratives.

Chapter 4: Results

Introduction

In this chapter, I present and discuss the results of this research. I also provide explanations of the results in respect to the statistical tests, which were performed while attempting to answer the research questions generated for this research. The purpose of this study was to assess the associations of Vitamin D and VDR gene polymorphisms and the risk factors for breast cancer causation among women in Texas, in the Southern United States. SurveyMonkey method was used in the distribution of survey questionnaires to the participants. Two hundred and fifty female participants consisting of 125 cases and 125 controls were recruited for this study. In the cases category, 75 women were premenopausal and 75 women were postmenopausal. Similarly, in the control category, 75 women were premenopausal and 75 women were postmenopausal. This was ascertained from the ages of the participants. The numbers were evenly distributed in both control and cases categories. The survey materials were mailed out to each potential participant, along with the informed consent forms. The questionnaires were on knowledge of VDR polymorphisms, breast cancer knowledge, and participants' response efficacy.

Research Questions and Hypotheses

The following were the research questions and hypotheses for this study:

1. Is there an association between VDR gene polymorphisms knowledge/awareness and decisions to reduce breast cancer risks?

$H_0 1$: There is no association between VDR gene polymorphisms knowledge/awareness and decisions to reduce breast cancer risks.

$H_a 1$: There is an association between VDR gene polymorphisms knowledge/awareness and decisions to reduce breast cancer risks.

2. Is there an association between knowledge of VDR gene polymorphisms and likelihood of mammogram screening?

$H_0 2$: There is no association between knowledge of VDR gene polymorphisms and likelihood of mammogram screening.

$H_a 2$: There is an association between knowledge of VDR gene polymorphisms and likelihood of mammogram screening.

The first research question "Is there an association between VDR gene polymorphisms knowledge/awareness and decisions to reduce breast cancer risks?" can be answered in the negative. This is based on a number of reasons. For example, the result of the first hypothesis indicated that knowledge/awareness of VDR gene polymorphisms does not predict people's willingness to reduce breast cancer by enrolling in breast cancer reduction programs (β = -**.076; t = -1.724; p >0.05**). In other words, enrolling in breast cancer reduction program is not a function of knowledge/awareness of VDR gene polymorphisms.

Also, the result of the second hypothesis indicated that knowledge/awareness of VDR gene polymorphisms did not predict likelihood of mammogram screening (β = -**.049;** $t = -1.19$; $p<0.05$). This implied that the likelihood of women to go for mammogram screening was not influenced by their knowledge/awareness of VDR gene polymorphisms.

Furthermore, the responses gathered from the respondents revealed that even though most of the women were aware and/or knowledgeable of the association between VDR gene polymorphisms and breast cancer, they did not enroll in any program to reduce breast cancer risks. The participants gave a number of reasons for their inactions. One of the reasons was lack of health insurance or inability to pay for treatment options. Another reason given by some of the women was that they lived in rural areas, where treatment programs were not available.

Additionally, some of the women believed in faith-healing, Thus, even though they were aware and/ or had knowledge of the disease process, they believed that their faith was sufficient to prevent any catastrophic event such as breast cancer from happening to them. In similar vein, some women believe that the God they serve would not let breast cancer kill them. Syncretism was another ideological belief system reported by the participants, which was why they did not enroll in breast cancer risk-reduction programs. They believed that syncretism could prevent diseases including breast cancer. Thus, even though they had some knowledge/awareness of any association between VDR gene polymorphisms and breast cancer, they were indifferent about the disease, because, they believed that it could not affect them in any drastic manner. This included some women who had already contracted the disease. For example, some women who were at various stages of breast cancer still believed that it would not kill them and/or that they could be saved through miracles. Thus, they were apathetic and/or nonchalant in enrolling in breast cancer risk-reduction or treatment programs. Therefore, $H_0 1$ should be accepted, while $H_a 1$ should be rejected.

The second research question: "Is there an association between knowledge of VDR gene polymorphisms and likelihood of mammograms?" can also be answered in the negative. A number of factors account for this. One of the reasons given by the participants was fear of the pain associated with mammogram. Thus, even though they were knowledgeable of VDR gene polymorphisms, and its risk factor with breast cancer, the participants were complacent about mammogram screenings.

Cost of mammograms was another factor dampening some women's inclination or desire to go for mammograms. Furthermore, some women were afraid that mammogram screenings might give them bad news of cancerous findings. Thus, they prefer not to know. Similarly, some women indicated that the reason they preferred not to bother about going for mammogram screening was that their husbands, boyfriends, or significant other might leave them, if mammogram detects cancer in them.

Furthermore, some women indicated that they were shy. Thus, even though they were knowledgeable of the risk factors, they would rather not go for mammogram screening, as they would not like to expose their breasts or any part of their body, which they considered as "private".

Also, even though some of the women had some knowledge/awareness of VDR gene polymorphisms and breast cancer, their general apathy about going for mammograms was due to fatalism. The individuals that held this belief assumed that breast cancer is beyond human control and that going for mammogram would not change whether they get cancer or not. For these reasons, some of the women delayed or avoided mammographic screenings, even though they had knowledge of the associative risk factors. Therefore, $H_0 2$ should be accepted, while $H_a 2$ should be rejected.

The foregoing can be stated as follows: Although these women were knowledgeable and/or aware of the probability that VDR gene polymorphisms could increase an individual's chances of getting breast cancer, most of the women were reluctant to enroll in breast cancer risk-reduction programs. Therefore, knowledge/awareness of the association between VDR gene polymorphisms and breast cancer did not necessarily influence individuals' decisions to reduce breast cancer risks. For these reasons, $H_0 1$ should be accepted, while $H_a 1$ should be rejected.

Thus, even though some people strongly agreed that it is beneficial to go for genetic testing and mammographic screenings, they still were reluctant to do so.

In respect to Hypothesis 2, it was observed that there were no associations between knowledge about VDR polymorphisms and breast cancer risks and decision to submit to mammographic screening among the participants. For example, although some of the participants were aware of the dangers implicit in getting breast cancer, some indicated they did not subscribe to going for mammograms, and some women were still unsure of whether or not to enroll in cancer risk-reduction programs.

Similarly, although some women strongly agreed that early cancer detections could save their lives, some women disagreed that early cancer detection could save anyone's life. Some of those who disagreed believed that fate or destiny controls a person's life. Therefore, they did not think it made sense enrolling in any programs. They believed that involving themselves in programs could not change whether a person dies from cancer or not. Such individuals, regardless of their knowledge about VDR gene polymorphisms and breast cancer risks, are not likely to submit to mammographic screenings. They are also not likely to make lifestyle changes to decrease their susceptibilities to breast cancer.

Basically, majority of the women who reported low rates of mammogram (or breast) screening blamed it on the unaffordability of mammograms, cultural beliefs or cultural influences, health beliefs, religious beliefs and sociodemographic characteristics. This buttressed the point that knowledge of a disease process may not necessarily influence an individual's decision to submit to mammogram screenings. Therefore, Null Hypothesis 2 could not be rejected. It revealed that there were no associations between knowledge about VDR polymorphisms and breast cancer risks and the individual's decisions to submit to mammogram screening. A number of reasons accounted for this, including apathy, fear of diagnostic outcome, and poverty (inability to pay for programs).

In order to answer the research questions, statistical analyses of the data were conducted. Statistical analysis was conducted, to help in the explanations of the characteristics of the participants. Also, statistical analysis helped to explain any associations or correlations between the dependent and independent variables used in this research. Furthermore, a linear regression analysis was performed in respect to the dependent variables used in this research (i.e., Vitamin D intake, either through direct sunlight exposure or through supplementation and periodic breast examinations).

Statistical Data Analysis

Statistical data analysis was used in comparing the variables and testing the hypotheses. The variables were tested through correlation and regression analyses.

Tables 3 to 12 below convey the results obtained through correlation analysis, and Chi-Square Tests. When the variables of interest were analyzed, it was found that, with a correlation coefficient of -.15 *and a p < .05,* there was a negative correlation between knowledge about VDR polymorphism and breast cancer risks and decision to submit to mammographic screenings. Thus, H_0 is retained in the second hypothesis as a unit increase in the knowledge of VDR polymorphisms did not translate to a unit increase in its influence to make the women submit to mammographic screenings.

Research question and Hypothesis One

Dependent Variable = Decision to reduce breast cancer (measured using an item that asked the respondents if they have enrolled in any breast cancer reduction program).

Independent Variable: Knowledge/awareness of VDR gene polymorphisms

Table 3

Correlations

			Know_about_VDRgenepolymorphi	Enrolled in Breast Cancer reduction program
Spearman's rho	Know_about_VDRgenepolymorphi	Correlation Coefficient	1.000	-.107
		Sig. (2-tailed)	.	**.090**
		N	250	250
	Enrolled in Breast Cancer reduction program	Correlation Coefficient	-.107	1.000
		Sig. (2-tailed)	**.090**	.
		N	250	250

Note: All the tests of association conducted above (Chi-Square, Spearman rho and Pearson correlation) show that there is no association between VDR gene polymorphisms knowledge/awareness and decisions to reduce breast cancer risk as the p-value in all cases were < 0.05. Thus there is no association between the dependent variable and independent variable.

Table 4

Case Processing Summary

	Cases					
	Valid		Missing		Total	
	N	Percent	N	Percent	N	Percent
Know_about_ VDRgenepolymorphi * Enrolled in Breast Cancer reduction program	250	100.0%	0	0.0%	250	100.0%

Table 5

Know_about_VDRgenepolymorphi * Enrolled in Breast Cancer Reduction Program Crosstabulation

Count

		Enrolled in Breast Cancer reduction programme		Total
		No	Yes	
Know_about_ VDRgenepolymorphi	Don't Know	6	9	15
	To a low extent	72	52	124
	To a large extent	54	30	84
	To a very large extent	18	9	27
Total		150	100	250

Table 6

Chi-Square Tests

	Value	df	Asymp. Sig. (2-sided)
Pearson Chi-Square	3.836[a]	3	**.280**
Likelihood Ratio	3.788	3	.285
Linear-by-Linear Association	2.948	1	.086
N of Valid Cases	250		

a. 0 cells (0.0%) have expected count less than 5. The minimum expected count is 6.00.

Table 7

Symmetric Measures

		Value	Asymp. Std. Error[a]	Approx. T[b]	Approx. Sig
Interval by Interval	Pearson's R	-.109	.063	-1.724	.086c
Ordinal by Ordinal	Spearman Correlation	-.107	.063	-1.703	.090c
N of Valid Cases		250			

Research question and Hypothesis Two

Dependent Variable = Likelihood of mammogram screening (measured using an item that asked the respondents if they are likely to go for a mammogram screening).

Independent Variable: Knowledge of VDR gene polymorphisms

Table 8

Knowl_about_VDRgenepolymorphi * Mammogram Screening Crosstabulation

Count

		Mammogram screening		Total
		No	Yes	
Know_about_VDRgenepolymorphi	Don't Know	7	8	15
	To a low extent	69	55	124
	To a large extent	51	33	84
	To a very large extent	17	10	27
Total		144	106	250

Table 9

Chi-Square Tests

	Value	df	Asymp. Sig. (2-sided)
Pearson Chi-Square	1.580[a]	3	**.664**
Likelihood Ratio	1.575	3	.665
Linear-by-Linear Association	1.424	1	.233
N of Valid Cases	250		

a. 0 cells (0.0%) have expected count less than 5. The minimum expected count is 6.36.

Table 10

Symmetric Measures

		Value	Asymp. Std. Error[a]	Approx. T[b]	Approx. Sig.
Interval by Interval	Pearson's R	-.076	.063	-1.194	**.233[c]**
Ordinal by Ordinal	Spearman Correlation	-.076	.063	-1.193	**.234[c]**
N of Valid Cases		250			

Note: All statistical test of association conducted on the second hypothesis also showed that there is no association between knowledge of VDR gene polymorphisms and likelihood of enrolling in mammograms as all the obtained *p*-value were < 0.05.

Summary of Linear Regression Analyses in Tabular Form

Hypothesis One

Table 11.

Linear Regression For Hypothesis One

Model	B	SE B	β	t	P
Constant)	54.14	2.165		25.003	.000
Knowledge of VDR gene pmp	-.070	0.40	-.109	-1.724	.086

Note: Linear Regression For Hypothesis One Shows result of how knowledge/awareness of VDR gene polymorphisms predicts decision to reduce breast cancer risk

Hypothesis Two

Table 12.

Model	B	SE B	β	t	P
Linear Regression For Hypothesis Two					
Constant)					
	.497	.069		7.248	.000
Knowledge of VDR gene pmp					
	-.049	0.41	-.076	-1.194	.233

Note: Linear Regression For Hypothesis Two shows result of how knowledge/awareness of VDR gene polymorphisms predicts likelihood of mammogram screening

Age Distribution

This is part of descriptive statistics. It was used to indicate how the sample (or participants) was grouped. The participants were categorized into six age distributions with intervals of nine, as follows: 1=20 to 29; 2 =30 to 39; 3= 40 to 49; 4=50 to 59; 5=60 to 69, and 6=70 and older. The youngest in the set of participants was 20 years of age, and the oldest was 70 years of age. The mean age was 45 years (SD=18.71), as shown in Table 13 below.

Table 13

Calculation of Mean and Standard Deviation with Respect to Age

Data	Data - Mean	(Data - Mean)2
≥ 20-year-olds	20 - 45 = -25	$(-25)2 = 625$
≥ 30-year-olds	30 - 45 = -15	$(-15)2 = 225$
≥ 40-year-olds	40 - 45 =-5	$(-5)2 =25$
≥ 50-year-olds	50 - 45 =5	$(5)2 =25$
≥ 60-year-olds	60 - 45 =15	$(15)2 =225$
≥ 70-year-olds	70 - 45 =25	$(25)2 =625$
Total = 270		Total = 1750
(270/6) = 45 (mean age)		Variance (1750) / (6-1) = 350
		Standard deviation = $\sqrt{(350)}$ = 18.71

Education Distribution

The educational levels of the participants, as shown in Table 14, ranged from those who did not complete high school to those who completed graduate or professional degrees. The educational variable was coded into five groups, with 1 representing *less than high school*, 2 representing *finished high school*, 3 representing *some college*, 4 representing *completed college*, and 5 representing *graduate/professional* educational level of attainment. The statistical mean was calculated as follows.

Table 14

Calculation of Mean and Standard Deviation in Respect to Education

Data	Data – Mean	(Data – Mean)2
Less than high school = 1	1 - 3 = -2	$(-2)2 = 4$
Finished high school= 2	2 - 3 = -1	$(-1)2 = 1$
Some college level= 3	3 - 3 =0	$(0)2= 0$
Completed college= 4	4 - 3 =1	$(1)2= 1$
Graduate/professional= 5	5 - 3 =2	$(2)2= 4$
Total= 15		Total = 10
(15/5) = 3 (mean education)		Variance (10) / (5-1) = 2.5
		Standard deviation = $\sqrt{2.5}$ = 1.58

Income Distribution Variable

The income distribution variable among the participants, Tables 15 and Table 16, ranged from $20,000 per annum to over $80,000 per annum. The statistical mean was 4.53, while standard deviation was 2.45 or mean 4.53 (SD=2.45). On average, the mean income of the participants was $45,000. The statistical mean was calculated as follows.

Table 15

Calculation of Mean and Standard Deviation with Respect to Income

Data	Data -Mean	(Data– Mean)2
Less than $20,000=1	1 – 4.5 = -3.5	(-3.5)2=12.25
Between $20,000-30,000=2	2 – 4.5 = -2.5	(-2.5)2=6.25
Between $30,000-$40,000 =3	3 – 4.5 = -1.5	(-1.5)2=2.25
Between $40,000-$50,000 =4	4 – 4.5 = -0.5	(-0.5)2=0.25
Between $50,000-$60,000= 5	5 – 4.5 =0.5	(0.5)2=0.25
Between $60,000-$70,000 =6	6 – 4.5 =1.5	(1.5)2=2.25
Between $70,000-$80,000 =7	7 – 4.5 = 2.5	(2.5)2=6.25
More than $80,000 = 8	8 – 4.5 = 3.5	(3.5)2= 12.25
Total= 36		Total = 42
(36/8) = 4.53 (mean income)		Variance (42) / (8-1) = 6
		Standard deviation = $\sqrt{6}$ = 2.45

Note: The statistical mean of 4.53 (SD=2.45) for income level of the participants revealed that on average, the participants were within the annual income bracket of ($40,000 + 50,000) / (2) = $45,000.

Table 16

Summation of Descriptive Statistics of Ordinal Demographic Variables

Statistical mean Standard deviation
Age: 45.0 (SD=18.71).
Educational attainment 3.0 (SD=1.58)
Annual income 4.53 (SD=2.45)

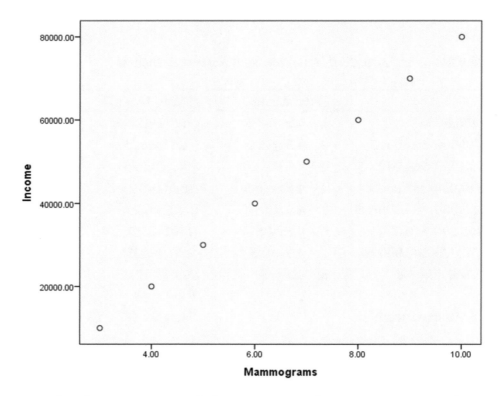

Figure 12. Graphical presentation of the association between income and exposure to mammograms.

Figure 12 revealed that there was a linear and proportionate correlation between income and mammograms. The graph indicated that women with higher income were more willing to submit to mammograms than women who earned lower income. For example, a woman might be knowledgeable of the disease process; yet, low income could prevent her from going for treatment. The assessment also helped explain why some women delay going for cancer treatments or enrolling in cancer risk-reduction programs (due to low or no income).

In the survey, some women indicated that low income was what curtailed their likelihood of going for mammograms. The survey revealed that women who had knowledge/awareness of VDR gene polymorphisms and risks of breast cancer were more likely go for mammograms, if they had higher income. On the other hand, women with lower income indicated lower inclination of going for a mammograms. This was probably because a woman with higher income can afford to pay, either directly or through her employment health insurance coverage. This option may not be available to unemployed or low-income women.

Demographic Data

In this study, 84 participants from Houston, 83 participants from San Antonio, and 83 participants from Dallas were surveyed. Table 17 presents a racial or ethnical breakdown of the participants from the three Texas cities of Houston, Dallas, and San Antonio. The majority of the participants (60%) were white females. The second largest racial group was women of Hispanic ethnicity, comprising 20% of the participant population. Blacks (of non-White, non-Hispanic ethnicity) made up 10%

of the participant population, while women of Asian/Pacific Islander descent comprised 8% of the participants. Native American women and those who considered themselves as "other" made up the remaining 0.8% and 1.2% of the participant population, respectively.

Table 17

Racial or Ethnic Characteristics of Participants

Race or ethnicity	Frequency	Percent
White (non-Hispanic)	150	60
Black (non-Hispanic)	25	10
Hispanic	50	20
Asian (and/or Pacific Islander)	20	8
Native American	2	0.8
Other	3	1.2
Total	250	100%

Next is Table 18, which gives a presentation of the responses obtained from the participants concerning their personal and family histories of breast cancer. Table 18 is also a portrayal of the participants' responses as to whether they and/or their family members had health insurance coverage. For example, 60 (24%) of the participants indicated that they had previous breast cancer diagnoses—whether benign or metastatic—in one of their breasts. On family history of breast cancer, 190 (75%) of the participants indicated that they had family members who had, at one time or another, been diagnosed with breast cancer—whether metastatic or benign. Also, 120 (48%) of those who responded indicated that they had a current or ongoing diagnosis of breast cancer. Equally, 130 (52%) of the participants indicated that their family members had current or ongoing breast cancer diagnoses. Furthermore, 180 (72%) of the participants stated that they had health insurance coverage, while 70 (28%) indicated that they did not have health insurance, but that their family members may have had health insurance during the time the family member was diagnosed with breast disease. The foregoing demonstrates that efforts to exclude individuals with histories of breast disease through questionnaire were abortive.

Table 18

Responses to Family and Personal History of Breast Cancer Demographic Variables

Relationship	Previous	Current	Health Insurance
Personal history of B/cancer?	60 (24%)	120 (48%)	180 (72%)
Family history of B/Cancer?			
	190 (75%)	130 (52%)	70 (28%)
Total	250 (100%)	250 (100%)	250 (100%)

Tables 19 and 20 show the statistical means and standard deviations for dependent and independent variables used in this study. These means and standard deviations were separately and individually calculated, based on the responses given by the respondents. Since these variables were not the same, they could not be measured on the same scale; thus, they were not summative and cannot be added together. From these tables, it can be seen that 75% of the participants had family members who had previous histories of breast cancer. This number was reduced to 52% (current) incidence, probably due to survival from breast cancer or mortality among the family members due to the disease. However, from the survey questionnaire forms filled out by the participants, only about 31% of the population revealed that they had mammograms within the past year. Also, only 42% indicated that they performed regular monthly breast self-exams. From the calculations, the statistical mean for mammograms was 49 (SD=21.82), while the statistical mean for breast self-exams was 56 (SD=29.2).

Knowledge of breast cancer risk factors, with a statistical mean of 66.37 (SD=31.15), signified that the participants answered about 66.4% of breast cancer risk factor questions correctly. Daily sunlight exposure had a statistical mean of 4.65 (SD=2.91). This shows that, on average, only 5% of the participants knew that exposure to sunlight is an important means of reducing breast cancer risks. Similarly, daily Vitamin D intake (through supplementation) had a low statistical mean of 3 (SD=1.58). This shows that only 3% of the population knew that Vitamin D can be obtained through dietary supplements.

The assessment of response efficacy was performed using Likert Scale type questions. The participants were asked, on a scale of 1 to 5, to indicate how important breast cancer screening was to them, how important Vitamin D was to them, and their resolve or determination to participate in recommended programs. The assessment contained five levels of responses ranging from 1 to 5 (with 1 representing *strongly agree* and 5 representing *strongly disagree*. The calculations were performed as seen in Table 19.

Table 19

Descriptive Statistics for Response Efficacy Using Likert Scale Type Questions

Participants were asked to indicate, on a scale of 1 to 5, their resolve and determination to engage in programs that could reduce breast cancer risks.

Do you agree that exposure to Vitamin D could help in reducing breast cancer?

Data	Data - Mean	(Data– Mean)2
Strongly agree=1	1 – 3 = -2	(-2)2=4
Agree =2	2 – 3 = -1	(-1)2=1

Neither agree nor disagree =3	3 – 3 =0	(0)2=0
Disagree=4	4 – 3 =1	(1)2=1
Strongly disagree= 5	5 – 3 =2	(2)2=4
Total = 15		Total =10
		Variance (10) / (5-1) = 2.5
		Standard deviation = √(2.5)
Mean = (15/5) = 3		= 1.58

As shown in Table 19, the mean for the knowledge about Vitamin D Receptor polymorphisms and breast cancer risks obtained from the sample was 3 (*SD*=1.58).

Result: The statistical mean of 3, which was obtained for level of knowledge of Vitamin D Receptor polymorphisms in respect to using exposure to Vitamin D to minimize breast cancer risks revealed that many women were not aware of the importance of using Vitamin D to reduce their chances of getting breast cancer. The standard deviation was 1.58. Response efficacy also had a statistical mean of 3 (SD=1.58. A mean of 3 and a standard deviation of 1.58 in respect to response efficacy also revealed low levels of the participants' willingness to participate in breast cancer risk-reduction programs.

Self-efficacy is an individual's judgment in respect to how well he or she would carry out any recommended or prescribed course of action to resolve a prospective negative situation (Bandura, 2004). Although it is a personal judgment call on how much effort to put into resolving a personal health problem, participants in this study did not measure well in self-efficacy questions. The poor attitude reflected on the low statistical mean of 4.15 (SD=2.26), as shown in Table 13. This further indicated that only 4.15% of the population made an effort to reduce breast cancer risks. The negative attitudes also reflected on the daily sunlight exposure with a statistical mean of 4.65 (SD=2.91), and Vitamin D intake with a statistical mean of 3 (SD=1.58), respectively.

The reasons for low amounts of sunlight exposure varied among the participants. Some were due to office work environment, with little or no exposure to direct sunlight. Yet, some claimed it was due to religious reasons in which women are required to wear *burqa* or full *hijab*, preventing them from exposing a significant portion of their bodies to sunlight. This could pose a significant health problem. For example, since a significant proportion of daily intake of Vitamin D is obtained through sunlight, individuals who shelter themselves from sunlight may be at risk for breast cancer. This could be one of the reasons some of the participants in this research had low Vitamin D intake. Daily Vitamin D intake through supplementation had a poor statistical mean of 3 and a standard deviation of 1.58. This indicates that only 3% of the participants stated that they took the recommended 600—800 IU of Vitamin D through daily supplemental means.

Table 20

Descriptive Statistics of the Dependent and Independent Variables

	Statistical mean	Standard deviation
Mammograms	49	21.82
Breast self-exams	56	29.2
Knowledge of breast cancer risk factors	66.37	31.15
Daily sunlight exposure	4.65	2.91
Daily Vitamin D intake (supplementation)	3	1.58
Response efficacy	3	1.58
Self-efficacy	4.15	2.26

Findings and Discussion With Evidence Support

Table 21 shows the age-adjusted breast cancer incidence rates in the San Antonio (Bexar County) region, Dallas (Dallas County) region, and Houston (Harris County) region. Of the three regions, Harris County (Houston area) had the highest breast cancer incidence, 76,107. Next was Dallas County (Dallas area), with breast cancer incidence of 45,412. The Bexar County region had an incidence rate of 32,982 (Texas Cancer Registry, 2014).

Table 21

Age-Adjusted Breast Cancer Incidence Rates in Houston-Harris, Dallas, and Bexar Counties

Region	Population at risk	Cases	Crude rate	Age-adjusted rate	96% Confidence interval
Houston city	115654	714	617.4	429.5	[423.8, 431.9]
Harris County	21351968	76107	356.4	425.0	[397.7,463.6]
Dallas County	12245092	45412	370.9	427.9	[421.9,428.2]
Bexar County	8952747	32982	368.4	393.8	[389.5,398.1]
Combined	42549807	154501	363.1	418.1	[415.9,420.2]
State	130468320	514385	394.3	415.2	[414.1,416.4]

Note: Age-adjusted rate is what would have occurred if the population under study had the same age. Thus, because they do not have the same age, this becomes an adjusted summary of breast cancer incidences across the wide range of age differences in the cities of interest. Adapted from "Age-Adjusted Breast Cancer Incidence Rates," by Texas Cancer Registry(https://www.dshs.texas.gov/tcr/).

Next is Table 22, which shows a continuous increase in breast cancer cases in Texas from 2010 to 2014. In the three regions of interest, Houston (in Harris County), had the highest burden of breast cancer. This was followed by Dallas (in Dallas County), and San Antonio (in Bexar County) came third. When these observations were compared with the crude ratios for breast cancer in the entire state of Texas, it was noticed that Harris, Dallas, and Bexar counties had the highest disproportionate burden of breast cancer than any other areas in the state of Texas. All together, these three regions (Harris, Dallas, and Bexar counties) had a higher rate of late-stage breast cancer than anywhere else in the state of Texas. This occurred more among the African American and Hispanic ethnicities than among the Caucasian subgroup. This problem could be due to a number of reasons, including not going for early mammograms, not doing proper breast self-exams, and delayed initiation into breast cancer treatment programs. This, in turn, could have led to the increase in mortality rates observed in these three cities compared to elsewhere. For example, as shown on Table 15, the Houston (Harris County) region had a highest death rate than Dallas and Bexar counties. The Dallas area came second, and San Antonio (Bexar County) came in a distant third.

Table 22

Age-Adjusted Breast Cancer Incidence Rates in the State of Texas

Year	2010	2011	2012	2013	2014	2010–2014
Population at risk	12721084	12931849	13142034	13349399	13588525	65732891
Total cases	14386	14161	14996	15182	15544	74269
Crude rate	113.1	109.5	114.1	113.7	114.4	113.0
Age-adjusted rate	113.9	109.2	112.6	111.2	110.7	111.5
95% Confidence interval lower	112.1	107.3	110.8	109.4	108.9	110.7
95% Confidence interval upper	115.8	111.0	114.4	113.0	112.5	112.3

Note: All rates are per 100,000. Rates are age-adjusted to 2000 U.S. standard population Age-adjusted rate is what would have occurred if the population under study had the same age. Because they were not the same age, an adjusted summary of breast cancer incidence rates across the age differences in the state of Texas was presented. Adapted from "Age-Adjusted Breast Cancer Incidence Rates," by Texas Cancer Registry. (https://www.dshs.texas.gov/tcr)

A number of strategies could be adopted to reduce breast cancer morbidity and mortality rates among the target population. For example, breast cancer educational classes could be held periodically to increase awareness of the importance of early mammogram screenings.

Additionally, some foods such as fruits and vegetables could be used to prevent or retard breast cancer progression. These may include foods rich in fiber such as whole grains, beans, and legumes. Low-fat milk and dairy products, soybean-based products, foods rich in vitamin D, and food spices rich in anti-inflammatory properties may also be helpful in reducing breast cancer incidence rates.

Sunlight promotes the synthesis of Vitamin D from cholesterol in human skin. However, during the winter months and early spring (October to May), the sun is not an adequate source of vitamin D, especially for people living north of the Atlantic. Perhaps this is why most people tested during the winter and early spring are usually low in vitamin D, thus increasing their susceptibility to breast cancer. This may also apply to individuals in Dallas, where the climate is colder than in San Antonio and Houston (where the weather is usually very hot).

To minimize their susceptibility to breast cancer, individuals living in such cold climates may have to increase their Vitamin D intake through some food items rich in Vitamin D such as cod liver oil, trout, ham, fortified milk, fortified yogurt, soy milk, almond milk, fortified cereals, orange juice, pork chops, sardines, fish roe, eggs, chicken, beef, codfish, cheddar cheese, mushrooms, salmon, mackerel, tuna, raw milk, and caviar. It is suggested that individuals should consume two of these vitamin D-enriched supplemental foods on a daily basis, in addition to getting as much sunlight as possible. Educating the target population on these simple measures could have a positive impact in reducing breast cancer incidence rates.

A review of Tables 23 and 24 will reveal that Harris County (Houston area), Dallas County (Dallas area), and Bexar County (San Antonio area) had the highest breast cancer morbidity rates when compared with other counties and other regions in the state of Texas. The reason is not certain. However, it could be attributed to the large population at risk for the disease. For example, Houston is the largest city in Texas, San Antonio is the second largest, and Dallas is the third largest. Consequently, these three cities are part of the most populous counties in Texas. Thus, the ratio of high population densities compared to other areas with lower population densities could account for why Houston (in Harris County), Dallas (in Dallas County), and San Antonio (in Bexar County) had the highest disproportionate burden of breast cancer.

Another point is that Houston has a large population of African Americans, whereas San Antonio has a large population of Latinas, and Dallas has more Caucasians. The African American and Latina American ethnic populations have the propensity to delay going for breast cancer testing as well as delay in participating in breast cancer treatment programs compared to their Caucasian American counterparts. Therefore, there was a need to educate the people on the importance of regular mammograms, proper ways of doing breast self-exams, and early involvement in breast cancer treatment programs.

Table 23

Age-Adjusted Breast Cancer Incidence Rate in Some Other Counties in Texas

Region or county	Population at risk	Cases	Crude rate	Age-adjusted rate	95% Confidence interval
Cochran	7701	-	-	-	-
Delta	13288	26	195.7	140.1	[89.2, 212.3]
Gray	54247	93	171.4	139.5	[111.5, 172.6]
Runnels	26257	53	201.8	139.0	[102.3, 186.0]
Camp	31979	56	175.1	137.8	[103.1, 180.9]
Erath	100373	139	138.5	136.3	[114.0, 161.7]
Collingsworth	7874	-	-	-	-
Parker	297114	466	156.8	134.2	[122.0, 147.4]
Morris	33177	61	183.9	133.1	[100.0, 174.4]
Wilbarger	33419	54	161.6	142.2	[97.9, 175.0]
Walker	141921	184	129.7	131.3	[112.4, 152.5]
Combined	747350	1158	154.9	135.2	[127.3, 143.4]

Note: Age-adjusted rate is what would have occurred if the population of interest had the same age. However, because the people that made up this study group did not have the same age, Table 23 presents an adjusted summary of the participants' age and breast cancer incidences in selected counties in the state of Texas. The data were used to compare breast cancer incidences in Harris, Dallas, and Bexar counties. Adapted from "Age-Adjusted Breast Cancer Incidence Rates", by Texas Cancer Registry (https://www.dshs.texas.gov/tcr/).

Most of the African American women and Latinas, especially those living in rural areas, did not have health insurance due to low income. Therefore, they were unable to obtain breast cancer screenings or enroll in breast cancer treatment programs. Another barrier is that those living in the rural areas faced lack of public transportation to mammogram screening centers, which are usually located in the urban areas. One of the strategies successfully used by previous researchers in resolving this problem was to provide breast cancer educational classes through the churches (Kelley, 2011; Mangum, 2016; Patz & Zanecosky, 2017). Civic centers, shopping malls, and schools and colleges are other avenues through which the masses are reached to educate and motivate them in regard to early breast cancer screenings. Soap operas, TV talk shows, and magazines such as *Ebony, Cosmopolitan, Buena Vida,* and *Mademoiselle* could be some other useful outlets through which to educate the target population about proper techniques for breast self-exams, the need for regular mammograms, and the importance of genetic testing for Vitamin D Receptor gene polymorphisms. These practices could help in early cancer detection.

Early detection is the key to better prognosis in breast cancer. For early detection, the participants were instructed to know the signs and symptoms to watch for. Thus, educating the target population on the risk factors as well as the early signs of breast cancer is essential, especially among African American and Latina Americans, because of their cultural beliefs and lack of knowledge about breast cancer. In this research, the early signs and symptoms of breast cancer that the participants were educated on included breast pain, chest pain, itchy breasts, upper back pain, shoulder and neck pain, changes in breast shape, size, or appearance, changes in nipple appearance or sensitivity, swelling or lump in the armpits, and red, swollen breasts looking like *peau d'orange* (peel of orange). Despite regular breast self-exams and mammograms, any inconsistencies or abnormalities in the regular size or shape of one's breasts should signal a visit to a primary care physician for biopsy and further diagnosis.

Table 24

Age-Adjusted Breast Cancer Incidence Rates in Dallas, Harris, and Bexar Counties, Texas

Region or county	Population at risk	Cases	Crude rate	Age-adjusted rate	95% Confidence interval
Dallas	12245092	45412	370.9	427.9	[423.8, 431.9]
Harris	21351968	76107	356.4	425.0	[421.9, 428.2]
Bexar	8952747	32982	368.4	393.8	[389.5, 398.1]
Combined	42549807	154501	363.1	418.1	[415.9, 420.2]
State	130468320	514385	394.3	415.2	[414.1, 416.4]

Note: Age-adjusted rate is what would have occurred if the population of interest had the same age. As the population under this study did not have the same age, an adjusted summary of the participants' age and breast cancer incidences in Bexar, Dallas, and Harris counties was presented in Table 24. Adapted from "Age-Adjusted Breast Cancer Incidence Rates in Dallas, Harris, and Bexar Counties, Texas," by Texas Cancer Registry. (https://www.dshs.texas.gov/tcr/)

As can be observed in Table 25 below, (60/125 = .48) or 48% of the participants agreed that they felt relaxed after doing regular breast self-exams. Only about 1/125 = 0.008, or 0.8% of the population, strongly disagreed about that. Similarly, 52/125, or 42% of the participants indicated feeling confident about doing regular breast self-exams, while 3/125, or 2.4%, strongly disagreed with that notion. Also, 49/125, or 39.2% of the population stated that breast self-exams could help them find cancerous lumps in their breasts. However, 5/125, or 4%, of the participants strongly disagreed with that idea. Furthermore, 50 women, 50/125 or 40%, strongly agreed that early detection of breast cancer could save their lives, while five women (i.e., 5/125 or 45) strongly disagreed on that. Some of those who disagreed stated that "Fate controls everything." They believed that a person could get cancer and die, if it were destined to happen, regardless of the person's actions or inactions. Nevertheless, 58 of the participants (58/125 or 46%) strongly believed that they would see their doctors if they found any lump in their breasts, but five women (3/125 or 2%) strongly disagreed with the concept.

Table 25

Participants' Responses to Benefits of Breast Self-Exams (n = 125 Cases)

Questions	Strongly agree	Agree	Not sure	Disagree	Strongly disagree
1. I feel relaxed after breast self-exams	60	58	4	2	1
2. I feel confident about breast exams	53	43	24	3	6
3. Breast self-exams can help find lumps	49	50	12	9	5
4. Early detection can save my life	50	56	8	6	5
5. I must see my doctor if I find lump in my breast	58	49	10	3	5

Table 26 is a representation of the responses obtained from the control category (i.e., women who did not have breast cancer. They indicated that they had no family members with history of breast cancer). They were pre- and postmenopausal (n = 125). Therefore, they ranged in age from 20 to 70. About 70/125, or 56%, of these women agreed that they felt relaxed after doing regular breast self-exams. Only about 3/125, or 2.4%, of the women strongly disagreed on that. Also, 82/125, or 66%, of the women indicated feeling confident about doing regular breast self-exams, while 2/125, or 1.6%, strongly disagreed with that idea. Similarly, 85/125, or 68%, of the control category stated that breast self-exams could help them find cancerous lumps in their breasts. However, 1/125, or 0.8%, of this group strongly disagreed with that assumption. Additionally, 50 women, 69/125, or 55%, strongly agreed that early detection of breast cancer could save their lives. On the contrary, about three women (3/125 or 2.4%) strongly disagreed with the idea. Some of the women who disagreed gave various reasons, similar to the case category, for doing so. All in all, about 90women in the control group (90/125, or 72%) strongly believed that they would see their doctors if they found any lump in their breasts; however, two women (2/125, or 1.6%) strongly disagreed with the idea.

Table 26

Participants' Responses to Benefits of Breast Self-Exams (n = 125 Control)

Questions	Strongly agree	Agree	Not sure	Disagree	Strongly disagree
1. I feel relaxed after breast self-exams	70	40	9	3	3
2. I feel confident about breast exams	82	30	7	4	2
3. Breast self-exams can help find lumps	85	32	5	2	1
4. Early detection can save my life	69	40	8	5	3
5. I must see my doctor if I find lump in my breast	90	21	7	5	2

Table 27 reveals participants' responses to questions in regard to benefits derived from performing regularly scheduled mammograms. For example, 76 (or 60.8%) of the participants indicated that they felt more relaxed after obtaining mammograms, compared to only one person (i.e., 0.4%) who strongly disagreed with the idea. An overwhelming majority of women (48.8% + 40.4% = 89.2%) agreed that there were some benefits to participate in scheduled mammograms. For example, 61women (61/125, or 48.8%) strongly agreed, and 50 (or 40%) agreed that early cancer detection could save their breasts from being cut off through radical surgical mastectomy. However, while a larger percentage of women believed that mammograms could help detect cancerous lumps and could help save their lives, only very few enrolled in programs to rectify or remedy anomalous breast health. Despite their actions or inactions when confronted with real-life breast problems, the majority of the women indicated that they felt confident and more relaxed after getting mammograms. For example, 66 women (66/125or 52.8%) of the sample population felt that mammograms could help in early breast cancer detection and thus could help save their lives. Nevertheless, a few individuals remained skeptical. Such individuals indicated that they were not sure, or that they disagreed, or that they strongly disagreed.

Table 27

Participants' Responses to Benefits of Mammograms (n = 125) Cases

Questions	Strongly Agree	Agree	Not Sure	Disagree	Strongly Disagree
1. I feel relaxed when I get mammograms	76	40	6	2	1
2. I feel confident after mammograms	76	40	7	1	1
3. Mammograms can help find lumps	56	53	12	4	3
4. Early detection can save my breasts from being cut off	61	51	6	3	4
5. Early detection can save my life	66	49	5	3	2

Table 28 is a presentation of the control group's responses to questions related to potential benefits accruing from performing regularly scheduled mammograms. For example, 91 (or 72.8%) of the women in this group indicated that they felt more relaxed after obtaining mammograms. Only one person in this category (0.8%) strongly disagreed with the concept. The majority of these women (72.8% + 18.4% = 91.2%) agreed that there were some benefits in going for scheduled mammograms. For instance, 95 individuals (95/125, or 76%) strongly agreed about it, and 20 (or 16%) agreed that early cancer detection could save their breasts from being cut off through radical surgical mastectomy. Even though a larger percentage of these women believed that mammograms could help detect cancerous lumps and could help save their lives, only very few indicated that they enrolled in programs to prevent breast cancer occurrence.

Table 28

Participants' Responses to Benefits of Mammograms (n = 125) Control

Questions	Strongly agree	Agree	Not sure	Disagree	Strongly disagree
1. I feel relaxed when I get mammograms	91	23	7	3	1
2. I feel confident after mammograms	92	23	6	2	2
3. Mammograms can help find lumps	91	21	6	4	3
4. Early detection can save my breasts from being cut off	95	20	6	3	1
5. Early detection can save my life	96	24	2	2	1

Summary

Breast cancer is a disease of unknown etiology. It affects both men and women but occurs more in women than in men. Because women are the most afflicted, this research focused more on the female breast disease. In the United States, breast cancer is the second leading cause of cancer deaths among women. This study focused more on three large cities in Texas (Houston in Harris County, San Antonio in Bexar County, and Dallas in Dallas County). Based on the data extrapolated from Texas Cancer Registry, these three cities seemed to have the largest populations at risk for various types of cancers, including breast cancer.

This study served as a tool and a vehicle through which the target population was educated on breast cancer risk factors. It discussed the importance of using Vitamin D in reducing an individual's susceptibility to breast disease. It also placed emphasis on regular breast examinations (mammograms, clinical breast examinations, and breast self-exams), which may help in early cancer detection, early diagnosis, and better prognosis.

African American and Caucasian women were the focus of this study. This helped in comparing the two ethnic groups and being able to determine which ethnic group is more predisposed to the disease. Narrowing my focus was helpful in identifying which ethnic group carries a disproportionate burden of breast cancer morbidity and mortality. This knowledge could be helpful in having further discussions, drawing conclusions, and making recommendations, as will be seen in Chapter 5, which follows. Chapter 5 starts with a discussion of the research findings in relation to the purpose of the study. Next, the research outcome and results are discussed. In addition to these, the research questions and the hypotheses are reviewed. Chapter 5 also discusses the implications for positive social change and the strengths and limitations of the study, and it closes with recommendations for action and a summary.

Chapter 5: Discussion, Conclusion, and Recommendations

Introduction

In this chapter, I discuss the research findings in relation to the purpose of the research. I also discuss the research outcome and results. Additionally, the research questions and the hypotheses are reviewed. Furthermore, the implications for positive social change, the strengths, and the limitations of the study are discussed. The chapter concludes with recommendations for action and a summary.

The purpose of this study was to assess the associations between Vitamin D and VDR gene polymorphisms and breast cancer risks among women in Texas, in the Southern United States. I assessed VDR gene polymorphisms and the risks of breast cancer among these target populations to fill the gap that existed. Previous researchers focused only on using diet and exercise to reduce breast cancer risks (Guyton et al., 2003; Harvie et al., 2013). However, I found that Vitamin D can be used to reduce breast cancer risks. I indicated the relevance of using pharmacogenetic testing to detect existence of any anomalous VDR gene capable of precipitating breast cancer. Additionally, I promoted the use of mammograms in early breast cancer detection.

There had not been any epidemiologic study on the triangular association between Vitamin D metabolism, VDR gene polymorphisms, and breast cancer risk at the individual level (John et al., 2011). This became the platform on which the current research was based. I wished to educate the target population about the importance of using pharmacogenetic testing for VDR gene polymorphisms. Furthermore, in attempting to fill the gap left by previous researchers, I introduced ways to reduce breast cancer risks through intake of vitamin D. I further encouraged regular breast examinations, which can lead to early cancer detection and better prognoses. Figure 13 below shows how to carry out breast self-examination.

Figure 13

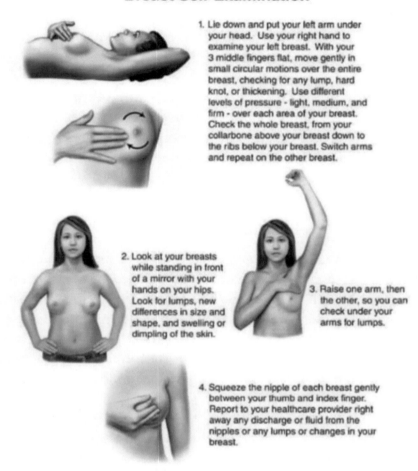

Figure 13: Breast Self-Examination
Public domain / Wikipedia

Research Questions and Hypotheses

The following research questions were addressed in this study:

1. Is there an association between VDR gene polymorphisms knowledge/awareness and decisions to reduce breast cancer risks?

$H_0 1$: There is no association between VDR gene polymorphisms knowledge/awareness and decisions to reduce breast cancer risks.

$H_a 1$: There is an association between VDR gene polymorphisms knowledge/awareness and decisions to reduce breast cancer risks.

2. Is there an association between knowledge of VDR gene polymorphisms and likelihood of mammogram screening?

$H_0 2$: There is no association between knowledge of VDR gene polymorphisms and likelihood of mammogram screening.

$H_a 2$: There is an association between knowledge of VDR gene polymorphisms and likelihood of mammogram screening.

Application of the Hardy-Weinberg equilibrium revealed the existence of a third variable (VDR-Ff) in the VDRs. This third variable was heterogeneous. Thus, it had the potential to generate free radicals, which could trigger oncogenes and lead to tumorigenesis. The first and second variables (VDR-FF and VDR-ff), however, were homogeneous. Thus, they were less likely to be oncogenic or tumorigenic. Therefore, the third variable (VDR-Ff), with its heterogeneity, revealed a high probability of generating VDR gene polymorphisms, thereby increasing risks of breast cancer.

Although these women were knowledgeable and/or aware of the probability that VDR gene polymorphisms could increase an individual's chances of getting breast cancer, most of the women were reluctant to enroll in breast cancer risk-reduction programs. Therefore, knowledge/ awareness of the association between VDR gene polymorphisms and breast cancer did not necessarily influence individuals' decisions to reduce breast cancer risks. For these reasons, $H_0 1$ should be accepted, while $H_a 1$ should be rejected. Thus, even though some people strongly agreed that it is beneficial to go for genetic testing and mammographic screenings, they still were reluctant to do so.

In respect to Hypothesis 2, it was observed that there were no associations between knowledge about VDR polymorphisms and breast cancer risks and decision to submit to mammographic screening among the participants. For example, although some of the participants were aware of the dangers implicit in getting breast cancer, some indicated they did not subscribe to going for mammograms, and some women were still unsure of whether or not to enroll in cancer risk-reduction programs.

Similarly, although some women strongly agreed that early cancer detections could save their lives, some women disagreed that early cancer detection could save anyone's life. Some of those who disagreed believed that fate or destiny controls a person's life. Therefore, they did not think it made sense enrolling in any programs. They believed that involving themselves in programs could not change whether a person dies from cancer or not. Such individuals, regardless of their knowledge about VDR gene polymorphisms and breast cancer risks, are not likely to submit to mammographic screenings. They are also not likely to make lifestyle changes to decrease their susceptibilities to breast cancer.

Therefore, Null Hypothesis 2 could not be rejected. It revealed that there were no associations between knowledge about VDR polymorphisms and breast cancer risks and the individual's decisions to submit to mammogram screening. A number of reasons accounted for this, including apathy, fear of diagnostic outcome, and poverty (inability to pay for programs). This was further exemplified in the study by Naqvi et al.(2016) involving 373 Pakistani women. Although the majority of the women knew the importance of early breast cancer detection, there was still general apathy and hesitation among the Pakistani women to participate in breast cancer risk-reduction program. The Pakistani women did not like giving responses to questions related to their breasts or other parts of their body. The Pakistani women thought it was sensitive, provocative, and embarrassing to respond to such questions. Perhaps this was due to cultural stigma and societal conservatism. For these women to respond positively, Naqvi et al. coined a phrase known as BCI. The program used web-based, self-administered surveys in assessing women's awareness, knowledge, and attitudes regarding breast cancer and early detection techniques. This was effective in getting Pakistani women to submit to the protocol. The general apathy among Pakistani women to engage in breast cancer risk-reduction programs, despite knowing the implications of not doing otherwise, was another indication that knowledge alone is not sufficient to induce compliance.

Additionally, in a study on breast cancer early detection among 7,066 Indian women aged 15–70 years-old and another research conducted among Indian nurses, Gupta et al. (2015) revealed poor literacy levels in respect to risk factors of breast cancer. Also, another research involving 441 Indian teachers found that, even though 36% of the participants knew about breast self-exams, they never actually performed it, and they never had any mammogram (Uwuseba, 2010). Although some of these women knew that delay in decisions to submit to mammographic screenings and make lifestyle changes could lead to deadly consequences, they were complacent about taking action to prevent disease occurrence. This further reinforced the idea that knowledge or awareness of a disease was not sufficient to make a person enroll in a risk-reduction program.

Deficiency in knowledge and lack of awareness about the risk factors for breast cancer can lead to monumental repercussions. For example, in Lagos, Nigeria, a breast cancer study found lack of knowledge about breast self-exams among nurses. The lack of knowledge resulted in only 8% of the sample size of 280 submitting to mammographic screenings in a 3-year period (Odusanya & Tayo, 2001; Uwuseba, 2010). Similarly, a study among Ethiopian nurses found that 42.2% of the nurses knew nothing about breast cancer, vitamin D, breast self-exams, and mammographic screenings (Lemlem et al., 2011).

Similar to the Nigerian situation, lack of knowledge prevented Ethiopian nurses from enrolling in breast cancer risk-reduction programs. This lends credence to Hypothesis 2, that there is no association between knowledge of VDR gene polymorphisms and likelihood of enrolling in mammogram screening. These women did not submit to the breast screenings because they lacked the knowledge. Japanese American women, however, regularly use breast self-exams, even when they have poor knowledge of its practice. This is because they believe that a breast self-exam costs them nothing, while mammographic screenings can be costly (Sadler et al., 2003). Thus, because of the high cost of mammograms, these women would not use mammograms, they would rather use breast self-exams.

However, in Selangor, Malaysia, Parsa et al. (2008) observed that 19% of the women practiced breast self-exams, 25% used clinical breast exams, and 13% practiced regular mammographic screenings. The research also revealed that Malaysian women engage in these practices because they are motivated and encouraged through their frequent visits to their family doctors. It is quite plausible that regular visits to their doctors bolsters their knowledge and awareness of the importance of regular clinical breast examinations. This notion partly buttresses the assumption in Hypothesis 2. In this case, there seem to be associations between knowledge about breast cancer risks and decisions to submit to mammographic screenings. For example, the Malaysian women who were in contact with their family doctors behaved differently than the Nigerian and Ethiopian women who had deficient knowledge on the use of mammographic screenings.

Cost is a significant barrier preventing Chinese American women from using mammographic screenings (Lin et al., 2008). This claim is in concordance with the observations made among Filipino American women. Research among these women revealed that Filipino American women in a higher socioeconomic income bracket are more likely to utilize mammogram screening than those in lower socioeconomic statuses. This lends credence that income influences a person's decision to go for or not to go for mammograms. Thus, even though the person is aware and has knowledge of the risk factors of breast cancer, poor socioeconomic status and/or lack of health insurance prevents them from using mammograms. Equally, costs prevent some women from enrolling in other breast cancer risk-reduction programs, thereby hindering them from making positive lifestyle changes. These claims are in accord with the observation made by Ham (2006) that low income and lack of health insurance hinders Korean American immigrants from using mammograms(or breast screening), despite their knowledge/awareness of its importance.

Lee et al. (2009) conducted a research study among 100 Korean American women. In that study, it was documented that only 51% of the women reported using mammograms. The study also found that even though mortality rate from breast cancer was on the increase, Asian women in the United States consistently reported low rates of mammogram (or breast) screening. This was blamed on cultural beliefs, health beliefs, and sociodemographic characteristics associated with individuals' mammographic screening experiences. This was further evidence that knowledge of a disease process may not necessarily influence an individual's decision to submit to mammogram screenings. Cultural influences, religious beliefs, sociodemographics, and affordability of a program should therefore be factored in when assessing a person's willingness to participate in a given program.

Review of Findings and Interpretation of Results

Roy's Adaptation Model (RAM) was the theoretical framework that guided this study. It was chosen because of its five concepts, which served as the backbone of this research. The five concepts are as follows:

- The health of the individual,
- The person (and her motivation, behaviors, beliefs, and attitudes),

- The health care personnel (nurse, physician) and readiness to educate and treat the person,
- The adaptation (willingness of the breast cancer patient to adapt and make changes—resilience, self-efficacy, and response efficacy), which could reduce risks for breast disease; and
- The environment (which includes modifiable factors affecting breast cancer such as mammograms, exposure to sunlight, dietary supplements, and the like).

RAM views an individual person in a holistic way. Its core concept is to help the person adapt. For this to happen, the healthcare system and its personnel must assume that a person is an open system capable of responding to stimuli from the internal and external aspects of the person (Roy & Andrews, 1999). Examining the outcomes of this study, while focusing on these tenets (or principles), makes it possible to evaluate the generalizability of the research result.

The Health of the Individual

The results generated from this study are not conclusive enough to determine how serious an individual is with respect to her health in general and breast cancer risk education in particular. This is due to a number of reasons. For example, the results obtained from this study revealed that knowledge and/or awareness of the disease process is not enough to make some women submit to mammographic screenings and make lifestyle changes. Not submitting to mammographic screenings and not making lifestyle changes does not imply that the individual is not serious about her health. Barriers such as cost of medical treatment, distance to healthcare centers, socioeconomics and sociodemographics, as well as cultural and religious beliefs are some of the hindrances that prevent most of these women from taking positive actions. For example, even though Korean American immigrants know about the deadly consequences of not enrolling in breast cancer risk-reduction programs, there are still low rates of mammographic screenings among them. These apathies, inactions or omissions could be blamed on cultural beliefs, health beliefs, and other uncontrollable sociodemographics.

The Person (and Her Motivation, Behaviors, Beliefs, and Attitudes)

A person's beliefs might be inimical to her motivation. This could pose a barrier as to the person's willingness and readiness to enroll in breast cancer risk-reduction programs. For example, some participants in this study believed that fate and genetics determine whether a person gets breast cancer or not. Those who held this view believed that a woman would get breast cancer if it was genetically based. In other words, if the disease runs in a woman's genes or family history, the person would get it, irrespective of personal efforts to prevent the disease. Those women therefore believed that fate controls everything and that, regardless of a woman's actions or inactions, commissions or omissions, she would still be afflicted with breast disease, if it were meant to be. This belief was held, not only by some of the less educated, but also by some of the most-educated participants in this study. Thus, fatalism influenced their decisions more than anything else.

By way of deductive reasoning, from the responses given by these women, it can be assumed that their fatalistic philosophy makes them surrender all hopes, events, or actions to destiny.

Thus, the fatalist generally sees herself as powerless to do anything beyond what fate brings to her. A person with this mindset will not likely do anything to reduce breast cancer risks. Another factor that negatively influences the minds of some women concerning their actions or inactions to enroll in breast cancer risk-reduction programs is due to the way breast cancer has regularly been presented to the public. For example, breast cancer has almost always been seen as a familial disease. In other words, breast cancer has always been referred to as a genetic disease that runs in families. Some women who already have developed a preconceived notion about the disease would not likely modify their behaviors such as smoking, excessive alcohol consumption, and sedentary lifestyle. Nor would they likely do anything to increase their Vitamin D intake. Similarly, the person would be less inclined to go for mammograms for early breast cancer detection.

The women who, due to fatalism, believe that even if mammograms could help in early detection of cancerous cells, but decide to do nothing to prevent the disease, need further education to realize that their belief is erroneous. Complacency, unresponsiveness, and inaction in regard to breast cancer can lead to nothing but catastrophe. Early detection of most cancerous growths, including breast cancers, can allow them to be surgically removed and the growth arrested and/ or reversed. Medical personnel and academia need to step in to help educate the masses on the importance of early cancer detection. Doing so could help change people's attitudes toward mammographic screenings. This is the centerpiece and the very significance of this study: to educate the target population through the dissemination of the research findings.

Patient education is part of the responsibilities shared by physicians and nurses. Educating the patient on disease control and prevention is as necessary as treating the disease. This is pivotal, not only in breast cancer prevention but also in the minimization of cancer metastasis. However, it must be noted that some medical school students and some nurses are grossly deficient in breast cancer knowledge. This assertion was buttressed through research findings among Angolan female medical university students (Sambanje & Mafuvadze, 2012), Nigerian nurses (Odusanya & Tayo, 2001; Uwuseba, 2010), Ethiopian nurses (Lemlem et al., 2011), and Indian nurses (Gupta et al.,2015). These medical personnel lacked the knowledge necessary to carry out efficient and effective services in their professions. For them to be able to educate the masses, they should have adequate literacy levels commensurate with their positions as nurses in order to make positive impacts in the lives of their patients, especially when teaching patients how to reduce breast cancer risks.

The adaptation (willingness of the breast cancer patient to adapt and make changes–resilience, self-efficacy, and response efficacy) can reduce breast cancer risks

Resilience

For the purpose of this study, resilience is defined as an attribute that measures an individual's ability to recover more quickly from a disease or any other difficult situations. With this in mind, participants in this study completed a questionnaire. The questionnaire was helpful in assessing the women's belief in regard to their level of resilience and quality of life in relation to breast cancer. In other words, the responses they provided through the questionnaires were used in assessing the ease or relative difficulty with which the individual could cope with the disease process if she were to be diagnosed with breast cancer. This research found out that individuals who are resilient have better coping mechanisms than those who are not. For example, I observed that breast cancer patients who were resilient had better quality of life than those who were not. In the current study, some participants strongly believed that remaining strong and resilient, even when diagnosed with breast cancer, could help their physical and emotional functioning. However, a few others strongly disagreed with the concept.

Self-Efficacy

Self-efficacy is an individual's personal judgment or belief of how well he or she can execute courses of action required to deal with prospective situations (Bandura, 2004). From the responses generated through this research, it could be inferred that 65% of the respondents would be able to exhibit positive coping mechanisms and positive behaviors if they were to be diagnosed with breast cancer. A person who has high self-efficacy and the resolve to overcome a negative situation would exert sufficient effort to actualize his or her other intents. Therefore, if self-efficacy were well executed, it could lead to successful outcomes in breast cancer situations. Conversely, a person with little or no self-efficacy may likely relinquish effort early when faced with adversities. Thus, without self-efficacy, a woman's effort and willingness to fight breast cancer may diminish, leading to disastrous consequences.

Self-efficacy affects every aspect of human life. Therefore, I thought it necessary to assess and determine the beliefs these participants held regarding their willingness to positively change an otherwise negative situation, such as breast cancer. The assessment made it possible to ascertain whether the women could actually withstand challenges competently. The assessment was also necessary in that it helped unveil what other treatment choices were available to breast cancer patients. This made it possible for concerned individuals to think about all available options ahead of time, rather than making the decision in the face of the challenges.

In the views shared by Mbeba et al. (2011) and Hung (2015), knowledge of a disease process can increase a person's self-efficacy and behavioral changes. Their views are not different from those observed in this study. For example, because an overwhelming majority of the respondents in this study positively responded by saying *strongly agree*, it is reasonable to conclude that knowledge in regard to using sunlight exposure and Vitamin D supplements to reduce the risks of breast cancer has a significant correlation with self-efficacy and response efficacy.

Response Efficacy

While self-efficacy is an individual's willingness to subdue an illness, response efficacy is an individual's belief as to whether a recommended course of action or step to be taken will actually avert or prevent the threat. For example, in this study, some of the women strongly agreed that adequate sunlight exposure and/or Vitamin D supplementation could protect them from breast cancer. Similarly, some of the participants strongly agreed that submitting to mammographic screenings could help in early breast cancer detection and diagnosis.

However, in research conducted among 290 Kuwaiti female schoolteachers, their knowledge, awareness, behaviors, and practices regarding breast cancer risk reduction were assessed (Alharbi et al., 2011). The study revealed an insufficient level of knowledge among these female teachers in respect to breast cancer. This became another instance where professionals registered low knowledge about the usefulness of mammograms and breast self-exams as tools for early detection of breast cancer. Additionally, the research among 100 Korean women (Lee et al., 2009) revealed that even though these women were knowledgeable of the consequences of not engaging in mammograms, they still abstained from it, thus further demonstrating that knowledge concerning breast cancer and how to reduce its risks cannot be associated with behavioral change to prevent the disease. This was also observed in this study. For example, some women indicated that they strongly disagreed with breast self-exams. They thought breast self-exams were "immoral", based on their religious beliefs. Thus, although they knew the implications of their omissions or inactions, they still failed to make lifestyle changes to reduce their chances of affliction with the disease. This further shows that knowledge about breast cancer and how to reduce its impact might not have any association with one's desire to change one's behavior and prevent a disease.

Additionally, in this study, there were some individuals whose religious beliefs encouraged wearing *hijab*. This garment covers a significant portion of a person's body, preventing the individual from exposure to sunlight. Therefore, even though the person is knowledgeable about the benefits of sunlight, she still would not alter her behavior to reduce the risks of breast cancer. Furthermore, due to religious beliefs, some women who attended faith healing churches stated that they would not take any medications, including Vitamin D supplements. Some also said that they would not submit to mammographic screenings. This further indicates that knowledge about breast cancer, and how to reduce the risks of breast cancer, is not enough to make a person alter their beliefs and behaviors. Nevertheless, individuals with a positive outlook, those with strong resolve, those with strong response efficacy, and those with strong self-efficacy, indicated that they would very likely participate in programs that could reduce their risks of getting breast cancer.

The Environment

The environment (rural, urban, suburban) where a woman lives or grew up in could play a role in what she believes and how she fights a disease. Environment includes modifiable factors affecting breast cancer such as place of habitation, personal beliefs, exposure to mammograms, exposure to sunlight, dietary supplements. For example, San Antonio, Texas, is predominantly inhabited by Hispanic Americans. Houston, Texas, is largely inhabited by African Americans, while Dallas has a larger population of Caucasian Americans. People who live close together have a tendency to influence each other's health beliefs and decision-making practices. This probably accounts for why women responded to the questionnaires in a way peculiar to each city. For example, whereas more Caucasian Americans from Dallas responded favorably to the use of mammograms, more African Americans in Houston indicated that they practiced breast self-exams, and Latinas in San Antonio practiced a mixture of both.

Syncretism, which is the mixture of more than one system of health belief or practice, can be observed in a community where people of the same ethnicity live together. For example, in Houston, Texas, Asian American women (Vietnamese, Korean, Japanese, Chinese), acknowledged the use of therapies that mixed acupuncture (or Eastern medical practices) with American or Western medical forms of breast cancer prevention and treatment. This was also true among some Nigerians, who claimed that they mixed voodoo or natural medicine (usually processed by a *dibia*, also referred to as a "native doctor") with Western medical formulas in their attempts to prevent or cure cancer. Similar claims were made by Afro-Caribbeans from Jamaica, St. Kitts, Antigua, St. Maarten, Saba, and Trinidad and Tobago, who indicated that they intermixed *obeah* (the Caribbean version of voodoo) and Western therapies in preventing or treating various diseases, including cancers. These beliefs and practices could delay seeking real medical treatment for such a dreadful disease as breast cancer, especially if the effectiveness of the syncretistic therapy is not verifiable. However, one thing is clear: Any delays in getting efficacious treatment of cancer lead to a detrimental outcome.

For example, women who practice these beliefs are likely to ignore clinical mammographic screenings. In the current study, there were women whose religious beliefs included faith healing—for example, Faith Tabernacle, Jehovah's Witnesses, The Church of Jesus Christ of Latter-day Saints (Mormonism). They believe that the God they serve would not allow breast cancer to afflict them. When asked what they would do if it occurred, common answers were "God forbid," or "God will deliver me from such an ailment," or "It is not my portion." Thus, some of those women gave *strongly disagree* as their response to any practices that could reduce their chances of getting breast cancer, including the use of Vitamin D supplements and mammograms. Some of the women even perceived breast self-exams as taboo or immoral. They indicated that they could not touch themselves. Such beliefs can lead to late-stage breast cancer diagnoses, poor prognoses, and deadly outcomes.

Implications for Positive Social Change

The implications for positive social change are as follow: This study could promote awareness of the importance of regular mammographic and pharmacogenetic testing for Vitamin D Receptor gene polymorphisms. It could also promote awareness of the risk factors for breast cancer and early detection, and it could lead to timely undertaking of appropriate therapeutic measures. Timely interventions can save lives. Delay can lead to death.

Furthermore, educating the target population in these areas could promote adequate intakes of vitamin D, reduce fear about mammograms, and decrease prevalence of late-stage breast cancer diagnoses. Thus, educating the target population could help in decreasing breast cancer morbidity and mortality rates in the areas of Houston, San Antonio, and Dallas, Texas, in particular, and the Southern United States in general. According to the Texas Cancer Registries (2017), the Houston, San Antonio, and Dallas areas have the highest at-risk populations. Breast cancer prevalence could be reduced with increased knowledge and awareness of the disease process.

The results of this study could have positive social change implications in other areas as well. For example, they could promote awareness among the target population regarding the importance of participating in regular mammographic screenings. The study could also increase the awareness of the at-risk population in respect to pharmacogenetic testing for Vitamin D Receptor gene polymorphisms, which, if ignored, can lead to oncogenes and tumorigenesis (cancer formation). Another perceived social change implication is that using Vitamin D to minimize breast cancer exacerbation is cost effective. Breast cancers, mastectomies, chemotherapies, and radiotherapies affect the self-esteem of cancer patients. These may affect individuals' perceptions and interpersonal relations; psychological well-being; and grooming behaviors, including hairstyle, style of dress, cosmetics, and outward appearance. Outward appearance is usually the manifestation of a person's inward disposition. In other words, a person's outward appearance is the primary focus of her identity recognition when it comes to making first impressions. Making first impressions matters; it depends on the way we carry ourselves and the types of messages we project about ourselves. These invariably affect the way others perceive or treat us. With this in mind, if pharmacogenetic testing for Vitamin D Receptor gene polymorphisms can be effective in identifying breast cancer risks, it is worth exploring. Also, if the application of Vitamin D can be effectively used in reducing breast cancer morbidity and mortality rates, the self-esteem of the target population could rise. This could augment or increase the social functioning of breast cancer patients. Their confidence in themselves could be restored or become reestablished. This would be especially true among those successfully treated with the regimen and those who could not otherwise have afforded regular cancer treatment. If this is an attainable positive social implication, then the purpose of this research is accomplished.

Human beings are social animals. We tend to be conscious of our surroundings. Also, we are often influenced by our social interactions and the impressions we give and receive from others. Thus, in women, the rate of the occurrence of altered appearances related to breast cancer treatments (i.e., mastectomies, chemotherapies) can reduce if hopes for breast cancer cure arise from serum Vitamin D augmentation, either through ambient sunlight exposure or through supplemental therapies.

Another social change implication related to the ones already discussed is that a woman's sense of belonging in areas of social functioning can be disrupted if she feels rejected by her peers or by the society of which she wishes to be a member. Such rejections can induce cognitive and behavioral setbacks. However, should application of Vitamin D and the reduction of the effects of Vitamin D Receptor gene polymorphisms be found as an effective antidote to breast cancer, the findings could help in ameliorating many negative setbacks due to breast cancer, reduce discriminations due to personal appearance resulting from mastectomy, and reestablish the person's acceptance by others. Another social change implication that could be derived from this research is that it might broaden the understanding of how cancer affects various races and ethnicities. This could make it possible to know how to individualize pharmacotherapy to treat various races or ethnicities in ways appropriate for their diseases.

Strengths and Limitations of the Study

Strengths

This study has some positive attributes or strengths. A significant strength is its use of self-administered questionnaires. Self-administered questionnaires made it possible for women in this study to fully express themselves without fear, duress, shyness, or intimidation. This is in contrast to the research of Naqvi et al (2016) among Pakistani women, where the authors conducted a person-to-person, descriptive cross-sectional study to assess the awareness, knowledge, and attitudes of 373 women toward breast cancer and early detection. It was found that Pakistani women were shy and hesitant to participate in breast cancer research and unwilling to respond to questions related to their breasts and other sensitive parts of their body. I used self-administered questionnaires in order to prevent similar embarrassments from occurring, and to reduce chances of stigmatization the women. A low level of education could be another reason why some women feel embarrassed about clinical breast examinations. In the current study, however, the majority of the women responded positively to both breast self-exams and clinical breast exams.

Another strength of this research is that it was possible to assess and understand various levels of self-efficacy and response efficacy. The research result, if well disseminated, could help clinicians in field epidemiology and in gynecological oncology to understand and determine why some individuals fail to make behavioral changes, even in the face of life-threatening adversities. An additional strength of this study is that the dissemination of its results could help future researchers to understand why some individuals have stronger and better self-efficacy and response efficacy than others. Yet, another strength of this study is that it taught participants (or concerned individuals) not to be judgmental of others, especially when attempting to determine why patients make decisions in peculiar or unusual ways. For example, a person who refuses exposure to sunlight might be because she is afraid of skin cancers (malignant melanoma, basal cell carcinoma, and squamous cell carcinoma, which are equally deadly), or for medical reasons (photophobia, photosensitivity) or religious reasons. Thus, in the face of adversities, it is necessary to empathize with individuals and try to understand why they make certain decisions. Understanding these could help healthcare policy makers to develop suitable pharmacotherapies for this population.

Limitations

One major limitation was the sample size. The study was based on a sample size of 250 participants drawn from the three largest cities in Texas (Houston, San Antonio, and Dallas). Although the participants were randomly selected through, a sample from just three cities could not be a true representation of the entire Southern United States. Also, a sample size of 250 participants could not be seen as a true representation of all women in the state of Texas, nor could it be seen as a true representation of all women in each of the three cities.

Even further, drawing samples from only the state of Texas could not be a true representation of women in the entire United States. Additionally, the three cities from which the sample was drawn have different climatic conditions. For example, Houston is in the southeast, and therefore hotter than San Antonio, which is in south Texas. Dallas is in north Texas, and much colder that Houston and San Antonio. This implies that participants from these three cities do not receive equal amount of exposure to sunlight. Therefore, these women do not have equal predispositions to breast cancer.

Similarly, ethnic groups are not equally represented in these cities. For example, whereas Houston contains more African Americans, San Antonio has more Hispanic Americans, while Dallas has more Caucasian Americans. As such, what applies to people in one city may not apply to those in another. Thus, it is fair to say that these environments are not the same, and the types of jobs worked by participants from these three cities are not exactly the same. For example, while Latinas in San Antonio may work more hours under the sun, Caucasian women in Dallas may more likely work long hours in offices and thus have less exposure to sunlight. This could be one of the reasons why there was a slightly higher breast cancer incidence in Dallas than in San Antonio. Perhaps the research would have had a different outcome if the sample had been drawn from only one city, one ethnic group, or one socioeconomic and sociodemographic stratum.

Self-administered questionnaires were used in this study. This method of information gathering had some limitations. For example, it was not possible to have face-to-face communication or interaction with the participants at all times to measure the accuracy of their responses. Similarly, using self-administered questionnaires made it impossible to visualize each participant to evaluate whether she was competent and of sound mind. Thus, the accuracies of the responses obtained through this mechanism could not be verified. These limitations could seriously affect the validity of the study.

To these limitations can be added yet another. Women who participated in this study ranged in age from 20 to 70. The earning power of these women was not the same. For instance, the older women might use Medicare, Medicaid, or other forms of health insurance to pay for mammograms and breast cancer treatments. These methods of paying for healthcare might not be available to younger women. This could make a difference, especially among unemployed or underemployed younger women who cannot afford mammograms or breast cancer treatments. Thus, it is not equitable to judge these different groups of women on the same scale of submitting or not submitting to mammograms. It was therefore not possible to determine the exact reasons participants in this study made certain health decisions. Thus, the results of this study cannot be perceived as an accurate reflection of what influences women to make behavioral changes in respect to enrolling in breast cancer risk-reduction programs.

Recommendations for Action

This study was undertaken to educate the target population on the associations between low serum vitamin D, Vitamin D Receptor gene polymorphisms, and the risks of breast cancer. Reducing the knowledge deficit in this area could minimize breast cancer risks among African

American and Caucasian women in the Southern United States and elsewhere. Social media, magazines, academia, and nurses and other healthcare personnel can be useful tools through which results of this research may circulate to the target population. Nurses should include culturally tailored interventions and individually specific approaches in attending to breast cancer patients. This is because the risk factors for breast cancer vary from person to person.

Patient-targeted outreach programs and the healthcare system navigation approach may be used in promoting mammographic screening and in encouraging women. This is particularly so among Nigerian, Angolan, Ethiopian, Egyptian, Indian, Pakistani, and Korean American women, in whose communities breast cancer knowledge is particularly deficient. With that said, further research is needed to unravel the interplay between acculturation, cultural factors, and health beliefs related to breast cancer screening behaviors among African American and Caucasian women in particular and all women in general.

To ameliorate these problems, educational outreach programs need to be established to help these women understand the risk factors for breast cancer. Helping the women understand the importance is not the only problem; they must also be granted greater access to mammography by reducing the cost and making it strategically available to those who need it. Doing so can facilitate early breast cancer detection and reduce mortality rates from breast cancer. Women who avoid exposure to sunlight, for a number of reasons, should be educated on the importance of obtaining Vitamin D through sunlight. However, those who cannot have direct exposure to sunlight due to medical reasons (photophobia or photosensitivity) should be educated on getting some Vitamin D through supplementation. This is particularly important, especially if it is not possible for the individual to change the behavior hindering her from increasing Vitamin D intake through exposure to direct sunlight.

The RAM theoretical framework used in this study has been successfully applied in numerous studies on how to minimize disease conditions and promote healing. However, it has not been extensively applied in breast cancer research. Nonetheless, because it contains five cardinal concepts or constructs relevant to health and disease prevention (i.e., the health of the individual, the healthcare system, adaptation, resilience, self-efficacy, response efficacy, and the environment), its application to the study of better ways to reduce breast cancer risks should be explored further. More importantly, healthcare workers and educators should learn strategies to encourage women to accept the guidelines about going for pharmacogenetic testing for early identification and diagnosis of abnormal Vitamin D Receptor gene polymorphisms. This, along with the use of Vitamin D and mammographic screenings, could lead to reduction in breast cancer incidence rates.

Recommendations for Future Research

Using diet and exercise to reduce breast cancer risks have been the precepts promoted by previous researchers (Guyton et al., 2003; Harvie et al., 2013). These precepts need to be reconciled with the notion of using Vitamin D as prophylaxis in retarding the progression of the disease, especially because research has shown that exposure to Vitamin D delays breast cancer progression.

The literature review revealed that there was no epidemiologic study which explained the triangular association between Vitamin D metabolism, Vitamin D Receptor polymorphisms, and breast cancer risk at the individual level (John et al., 2011). This became the ground from which the current research was developed. It is worth noting that future researchers can use this study as a template for validating the need to promote genetic testing for Vitamin D Receptor gene polymorphisms. This can also serve as a base for future researchers to validate the practice of using Vitamin D in reducing the risks for breast cancer and in promoting mammographic screenings as a means of early breast cancer detection among various populations of interest.

The three cities from which the sample was drawn (Houston, San Antonio, and Dallas) are culturally diverse. The populations in these cities comprise African Americans, Caribbean Americans, Caucasian Americans, Hispanic Americans, Asian Americans, and others. Breast cancer researchers should be aware of such diversity. Being cognizant of these ethnic diversities might enable breast cancer researchers to pay attention to diversity in women's attitudes, behaviors, and reactions toward any recommended programs such as breast self-exams, mammograms, sunlight exposure, and Vitamin D therapy. In other words, having an in-depth understanding of various ethnic groups and their cultures might enable future researchers to develop appropriate intervention protocols specifically tailored to resolve health problems based on ethnicity. From an ethnic difference perspective, this is crucial, because a number of abnormal Vitamin D Receptors have been suspected to increase breast cancer incidence rates among some ethnic groups but not in others. For example, whereas some researchers tie FokI (VDR-FF or ff or Ff allele) polymorphisms to the increase in breast cancer risks among African Americans, other researchers have different views or even see the findings as inconclusive (Shan et al., 2014). Further studies are needed in most of these areas, especially the areas that had been declared inconclusive.

In research involving breast cancer and human genetics, there have always been inconsistent and inconclusive research outcomes. For example, some researchers found no significant association between Vitamin D Receptor gene polymorphisms Fok1, Bsm1, Taq1, Apa1 and breast cancer risk in the Caucasian ethnic subgroup (Lu, Jing, & Suzhan, 2016). However, others believe that the same polymorphic alleles increase the risks of breast cancer in African American and Caucasian American women, but not among Latinas, American Indians, or Asian Americans (Abd-Elsalam et al., 2015; Gallicchio et al., 2015; McKay et al., 2009). It is possible that previous researchers may have looked at only two homogeneous aspects of Vitamin D Receptors, such as the Fok1 VDRFF and the Fok1 VDRff. The FF or AA and the ff or aa represent p^2 and q^2, respectively, of the Hardy-Weinberg Equilibrium. Both p^2 and q^2 are homogeneous. Thus, they cannot harbor free radicals, which can cause cancer. However, a third variable exists (2pq), which can harbor cancerous oxidants. This can be represented by VDRFf or Ff, or Aa. This is heterogeneous. Heterogeneity is usually a harbinger of cancerous growth. There has not been any documented proof that this third variable has been researched as a potential risk factor for breast cancer. The possibility exists, given the fact that genetic cellular heterogeneity promotes disharmony, reduces apoptosis, and can harbor free radicals. Free radical cells can form breast cancer. Future researchers should look into this exhaustively.

The differences in research findings could be due to sample sizes usually adopted in researches, the environments where the research was conducted, and many other variables. For future researchers to obtain better and more realistic outcomes, the causes of these ambiguities need to be deciphered and normalized. Additionally, as Vitamin D Receptor gene polymorphisms have been implicated in breast cancers among African American and Caucasian American women, this research study can serve as a clarion call for further assessments and more research on ways to promote the level of knowledge and awareness among these ethnic populations. Awareness of the disease process and an increase in knowledge on how to reduce breast cancer prevalence can increase women's confidence, resilience to fight breast cancer, response efficacy, and self-efficacy. The aim should be to help women prevent, cope with, and survive breast cancer.

Summary and Conclusion

Breast cancer is the major cause of death among women, not only in the United States, but also around the world. In the United States, it was estimated that about 266,120 new cases of invasive breast cancer and 63,960 new cases of noninvasive (*in situ*) breast cancer would be diagnosed in women in 2018. This was significantly higher than the estimate for 2017, which stated that about 252,710 women would be diagnosed with invasive breast cancer and about 63,410 women would be diagnosed with noninvasive breast cancer in the United States. Further, the number of deaths due to breast cancer in the United States was projected to be around 41,070 in 2017. However, the 2018 number of projected breast cancer-related deaths in women in the United States was 40,920. This is slightly lower than the 2017 estimate. Thus, it varies every year.

Breast cancer is a multifactorial disease. It involves both genetic and environmental risk factors. It has been postulated that breast cancer risks can be reduced through exposure to vitamin D. Also, Vitamin D has been known to modulate human biological processes, including immune response, bone metabolism, and cell growth regulation. When the growth of any cell can no longer be regulated, it results in cancer. Serum Vitamin D reduces uncontrollable cell growth. Therefore, it is possible that Vitamin D can protect against various cancers, including breast cancer. Because this is still a new area of research, results are emerging and thoughts are evolving about using Vitamin D in cancer therapies. Thus, the mechanism through which Vitamin D achieves its protective function is not well understood. Therefore, more research is needed in this area.

However, hope is still rising, as there have been some clinical indications that Vitamin D regulates cell growth. If so, then Vitamin D can be an essential modulator of apoptosis and cell differentiation. With these in mind, serum Vitamin D can help in suppressing cancerous growths. Based on these assumptions, one can postulate that Vitamin D can suppress or delay cancer cells from invading nearby cells and inhibit uncontrollable angiogenesis and cancer metastasis. Vitamin D can achieve this process through its Receptor identified as the p53 target gene. However, abnormal Vitamin D Receptors can create polymorphisms and promote breast cancer.

This quantitative, quasi-experimental study assessed the associations between Vitamin D Receptor gene polymorphisms (FokI and BsmI) and the risks for breast cancer among African American and Caucasian American women. In this study, time and resources did not allow for extensive direct experimentation, which could span for years. Therefore, its nature did not permit a direct observation of all the assumptions made.

In almost all aspects of research endeavors pertaining to human health, a number of legal and ethical issues always crop up, and breast cancer research is no different. The legal and ethical issues may vary depending on the nature and area of research focus. In breast cancer research, for example, ethical concerns may arise when screening patients for participation in the research. Similarly, ethical issues may arise during diagnosis and when treating those actually diagnosed with the disease. For example, obtaining or not obtaining patient, guardian, or parental consent may pose ethical concerns. To avoid such problems, this study only employed women who had reached legal age, between 20 years of age and 76 years of age. Also, the participants had to sign a consent form.

In this study, it was noted that some religions practice faith healing. In epidemiologic and clinical practice, this may pose a significant problem. For example, when a patient is not of legal age to sign a consent form for breast cancer treatment, and her legal guardians refuse to consent to the treatment, this may delay treatment before any legal battle is adjudicated or decided. In the meantime, the cancer may continue to spread. Future researchers should find ways to reduce such administrative and judicial protocols, in order to save lives.

Another area of ethical concern is when or how to seek reimbursements for therapies that some insurance companies deem to be experimental, such as high-dose chemotherapies, autologous bone marrow transplants, or off-label drugs. Future researchers should find a middle ground to accommodate cancer patients so that they may continue receiving treatments while reimbursement issues are settled.

Future researchers need to devise plans to deal with these types of ethical concerns in order to minimize delays that could exacerbate disease progression. When screening patients for diagnosis using mammography, the patient's best interest should be the focus; cost should not be the yardstick with which to measure the types of services rendered to the patients. When life is at stake, it becomes necessary to carry on with any process that could save lives. Such decisions should override every other decision, such as waiting for administrative protocols, waiting for health insurance verifications, and parental or guardian consent. Furthermore, future researchers should explore other methods of paying for essential treatment regimens in situations where a treatment modality is found to be potent and insurance companies happen to be delaying approval. Taking these steps may also save lives.

Additionally, future researchers should devise means to encourage women to periodically go for mammographic screenings. However, it is difficult to convince some women on the importance. This could be because some women are either shy about going through the process, or they may be afraid of receiving a negative health report. They thus prefer not to bother with going for a mammogram or treatment. This problem can be minimized by promoting breast cancer awareness programs through seminars, public speeches, and by strategically displaying posters, flyers, banners, and billboards. Beneficial results can also be achieved by conducting and holding conferences and press releases where and when possible. Television programs, soap operas, talk shows, church bulletins, and women's magazines such as *Ebony, Vogue, Cosmopolitan, Buena Vida,* and *Mademoiselle* could be good resources for disseminating messages about breast cancer risks. This strategy can help in reducing breast cancer incidence. How to resolve the problem of lack of funds for breast cancer research is another issue that future researchers should find ways to mitigate. Neither previous researchers nor this researcher have adequately addressed these concerns.

References And Resources For Further Reading

Abbas, S., Nieters, A., Linseisen, J., Slanger, T., Kropp, S., Mutschelknauss, E. J., . . . Chang-Claude, J. (2008). Vitamin D Receptor gene polymorphisms and haplotypes and postmenopausal breast cancer risk. *Breast Cancer Research, 10*(2), R31. doi:10.1186/bcr1994

Abd-Elsalam, E. A., Ismaeil, N. A., & Abd-Alsalam, H. S. (2015). Vitamin D receptor gene polymorphisms and breast cancer risk among postmenopausal Egyptian women Tumour Biol. 2015 Aug;36(8):6425-31. doi: 10.1007/s13277-015-3332-3. Epub 2015 Mar 25.

Acheson, L. S.,Lynn, A., & Wiesner, G. L. (2009). Self-administered, web-based screening of family history of cancer as a method to select appropriate patients for genetic assessment. *Cancer Research,(69)*2,Supplement January 2009. Retrieved from http://cancerres.aacrjournals.org/content/69/2_Supplement/1096.short doi:10.1158/0008-5472.SABCS-1096.

Alharbi, N. A., Alshammari, M. S.,Almutairi, B. M.,Makboul, G., & El-Shazly, M. K. (2011). Knowledge, awareness, and practices concerning breast cancer among Kuwaiti female school teachers. *Alexandria Journal of Medicine, 48*(1), 75–82.

Allahverdipour, H., Asghari-Jafarabadi, M., & Emami, A. (2011). Breast cancer risk perception, benefits of and barriers to mammography adherence among a group of Iranian women. *Women& Health, 51*(3), 204–19. doi:10.1080/03630242.2011.564273

Aluko, J. O., Ojelade, M. F., Sowunmi, C. O., & Oluwatosin, O. A. (2014). Awareness, knowledge and practices of breast cancer screening measures among female postgraduate students of a Nigerian federal university: Across-sectional study. *African Journal of Medicine and Medical Sciences, 43*, 79–86.Retrieved from https://www.ncbi.nlm.nih.gov/pmc/articles/PMC4682918/

American Cancer Society. (2010). Breast cancer early detection and diagnosis. Retrieved fromwww.cancer.org/cancer/breastcancer/index

American Cancer Society. (2013). Breast cancer risk and prevention. Retrieved from www.cancer.org

American Cancer Society. (2015). *Cancer Facts & Figures 2015*. Retrieved from www.cancer.org/research/cancer-facts-statistics/all-cancer-facts-figures/cancer-facts-figures-2015.html

American Cancer Society. (2017). *Cancer Facts & Figures*. Retrieved from www.cancer.org/content/dam/cancer-org/research/cancer-facts-and-statistics/breast-cancer-facts-and-figures/breast-cancer-facts-and-figures-2017-2018.pdf

American Cancer Society. (2018). *Current year estimates for breast cancer*. Retrieved fromwww.cancer.org/cancer/breast-cancer/about/how-common-is-breast-cancer.html

Amundadottir, L. T., Sulem, P., Gudmundsson, J., Helgason, A., Baker, A., Agnarsson, B. A., & Stefansson, K. (2006). A common variant associated with prostate cancer in Caucasian and African populations. *Nature Genetics, 38*(6), 652–658. doi:10.1038/ng1808

Anderson, L. N., Cotterchio, M., Vieth, R., &Knight, J. A. (2010). Vitamin Dand calcium intakes and breast cancer risk in pre- and postmenopausal women. *American Journal of Clinical Nutrition,91*(6),1699–707. doi:10.3945/ajcn.2009.28869.

Armistead, T. W. (2014). Resurrecting the third variable: A critique of Pearl's causal analysis of Simpson's paradox. *The American Statistician, 68*(1), 1–7. doi:10.1080/00031305.2013.8 07750 110

Azizi, E., Pavlotsky, F., Vered, I., & Kudish, A. I. (2009). Occupational exposure to solar UVB and seasonal monitoring of serum levels of 25-Hydroxy Vitamin D3: A case control study. *Photochemistry and Photobiology, 85,* 1240–1244. Retrieved from journals.plos. org/plosone/article?id=10.1371/journal.pone.0065785

Babbie, E. R. (2010). *The practice of social research* (12thed.). Belmont, CA: Wadsworth Cengage.

Beaudreau, S. A. (2006). Qualitative variables associated with older adults' compliance in a Tai Chi group. *Clinical Gerontology,30,* 99–107.Retrieved from internal-pdf:// Beaudreau-3280537102/Beaudreau.pdf

Berlanga-Taylor, A. J., & Knight, J. C. (2014). An integrated approach to defining genetic and environmental determinants for major clinical outcomes involving vitamin D. *Molecular Diagnosis & Therapy, 18*(3), 261–272.doi:10.1007/s40291-014-0087-2

Berry, D. A., Cronin, K. A., Plevritis, S. K., Fryback, D. G., Clarke, L., Zelen, M.,. . . Feuer, E. J. (2015), Effect of screening and adjuvant therapy on mortality from breast cancer. *New England Journal of Medicine, 353*(17),1784–1792. doi:10.1056/NEJMoa050518

Blanchard, C. M., Reid, R. D., Morrin, L. I., McDonnell, L., McGannon, K., Rhodes, R. E., & Edwards, N. (2009). Does protection motivation theory explain exercise intentions and behavior during home-based cardiac rehabilitation? *Journal of Cardiovascular Cardiopulmonary Rehabilitation and Prevention, 29*(3), 188–192.

Bolek-Berquist, J., Elliott, M. E., Gangnon, R. E., Gemar, D., Engelke, J., Lawrence, S. J., & Hansen, K. E. (2009). Use of a questionnaire to assess Vitamin Dstatus in young adults. *Public Health Nutrition, 12*(2), 236–243. doi:10.1017/S136898000800356X

Breastcancer.org. (2016). U. S. Breast Cancer Statistics. Retrieved fromwww.breastcancer.org/ symptoms/understand_bc/statistics

Buhler, V. (1988). *Vademecum for vitamin formulations.* London: Medpharm.

Buhler, V. (2001). *Vademecum for vitamin formulations.* Stuttgart: Wissenschaftliche Verlagsgesellschaft

Burkholder, G. J. (2014). *The absolute essentials of sample size analysis or: you too can be a statistical power guru.* Retrieved from PowerPoint Presentation College of Health Sciences, Walden University Libraries.

Cancer.net. (2017). *Cancer types: Breast cancer statistics.* Retrieved from http://www.cancer.net/cancer-types/breast-cancer/statistics

Cancer Research UK. (2015). *Why is early diagnosis important?* Retrieved from http://www.cancerresearchuk.org/health-professional/cancer-statistics/statistics- by-cancer-type/breast-cancer/survival#By

Carolinathermascan.com. (2013). *Breast cancer prevention: Facts & perspectives* Retrieved from http://www.carolinathermascan.com/breast-cancer-prevention--facts--perspectives.html

Centers for Disease Control and Prevention. (2011). *Healthy People* – HP2010 Final Review. Retrieved from http://www.cdc.gov/nchs/healthy-people/hp2010/hp2010-final-review.htm

CDC (2014). Death rates by race/ethnicity and sex. Retrieved from https://www.cdc.gov/cancer/dcpc/data/race.htm

CDC (2015). Breast cancer rates by race and ethnicity. Retrieved from http://www.cdc.gov/cancer/breast/statistics/race.htm

CDC. (2015). Breast cancer statistics. Retrieved fromhttp://www.cdc.gov/cancer/breast/statistics/

CDC. (2016). *Five-year summary: January 2011 to December 2015.* National Breast and Cervical Cancer Early Detection Program (NBCCEDP). Retrieved from https://www.cdc.gov/cancer/nbccedp/data/summaries/national aggregate.htm

Chang, B., Zheng, L. S., Isaacs, D. S., Wiley, E. K., Turner, A., Li, G., . . . Xu, J. (2004).A polymorphism in the CDKN1B gene is associated with increased risk of hereditary prostate cancer. *Cancer Research, 64*(6), 1997–1999. doi:10.1158/0008-5472.can-03-2340

Chang, B. L., Spangler, E., Gallagher, S., Haiman, C. A., Henderson, B., Isaacs, W., . . . Rebbeck, T. R. (2011). Validation of genome-wide prostate cancer associations in men of African descent. *Cancer Epidemiology Biomarkers and Prevention, 20*(1), 23–32. doi:10.1158/1055-9965.EPI-10-0698

Chen, L., & Li, C. I.(2015). Racial disparities in breast cancer diagnosis and treatment by hormone Receptor and HER2 status. *Cancer Epidemiology, Biomarkers & Prevention, 24*(11), 1666-1172. doi:10.1158/1055-9965.EPI- 15-0293

Chen, P., Hu, P., Xie, D., Qin, Y., Wang, F., & Wang, H. (2010). Meta-analysis of vitamin D, calcium and the prevention of breast cancer. *Breast Cancer Research and Treatment, 121*(2), 469–477.

Chen, S. J., Kung, P. T., Huang, K. H., Wang, Y. H., &Tsai, W. C. (2015). Characteristics of the delayed or refusal therapy in breast cancer patients: A longitudinal population-based study in Taiwan. *PLoS ONE, 10(6).* doi:10.1371/journal.pone.0131305

Chen, W. Y., Berone-Johnson, E. R., Hunter, D. J., Willett W. C.,& Hankinson, S. E. (2015). Associations between polymorphisms in the Vitamin D Receptor and breast cancer risk. *Cancer Epidemiology, Biomarkers & Prevention, 14*(10), 2335-2339.

Chlebowski, R., T., Johnson, K. C., Kooperberg, C., Pettinger, M., Wactawski-Wende, J., Rohan, T., . . .,Hubbell, F. A. (2008).Calcium plus Vitamin D supplementation and the risk of breast cancer. *Journal of the National Cancer Institute,100*(22):1581–1591. doi:10.1093/jnci/djn360

Colombini, A., Brayda-Bruno, M., Lombardi, G., Croiset, S. J., Ceriani, C., Buligan, C., . . .Cauci, S. (2016). BsmI, ApaI and TaqI polymorphisms in the Vitamin D Receptor gene(VDR) and association with lumbar spine pathologies: An Italian case-control study. *PLoS ONE, 11*(5). doi:10.1371/journal.pone.0155004

Creswell, J. W. (2009). *Research design: Quantitative, qualitative, and mixed methods approaches.* Thousand Oaks, CA: Sage Publications.

Crew, K. D. (2013). Vitamin D: Are We Ready to Supplement for Breast Cancer Prevention and Treatment? Retrieved from http://www.hindawi.com/journals/isrn/2013/483687/

Crew, K. D., Shane, E., Cremers, S., McMahon, D. J., Irani, D. & Hershman, D. L. (2009) .High prevalence of Vitamin D deficiency despite supplementation in premenopausal women with breast cancer undergoing adjuvant chemotherapy. *Journal of Clinical Oncology, 27*(13), 2151–2156. doi:10.1200/JCO.2008.19.6162

Dana-Faber Cancer Institute. (2017). *Turning point.* Retrieved from https://www.dana-farber.org

Darnell, J. S., Chang, C. H., & Calhoun, E. A. (2006). Knowledge about breast cancer and participation in a faith-based breast cancer program and other predictors of mammography screening among African American women and Latinas. Health *Promotion Practice, 7*(3 Suppl). doi:10.1177/1524839906288693

Deeb, K. K.,Trump, D. L.,&Johnson, C. S. (2007). Vitamin D signaling pathways in cancer: Potential for anticancer therapeutics. *Nature Reviews Cancer, 7*(9), 684–700.

Doheny,K.(2012).*African American women:Breast cancer more deadly?*Retrieved from https://www.webmd.com/breast-cancer/news/20121028/breast-cancer-african-american-women#1

Domenighetti, G., D'Avanzo, G., Egger, M., Berrino, F., Perneger, T., Mosconi, M., & Zwahlen, M. (2003). Women's perception of the benefits of mammography screening: Population-based survey in four countries. *International Journal of Epidemiology, 32*(5), 816–821. https://doi.org/10.1093/ije/dyg257

Engel, L. S., Orlow, I., Sima, C. S., Satagopan, J., Mujumdar, U., Roy, P., . . .Alavanja, M. C. (2013). Vitamin D Receptor gene haplotypes and polymorphisms and risk of breast cancer: A nested case-control study. *Cancer Epidemiology, Biomarkers, and Prevention,21*(10), 1856–1856.doi:10.1158/1055-9965.EPI-12-0551

Engel, P., Fagherazzi, G., Mesrine, S., Boutron-Ruault, M. C., &Clavel-Chapelon, F. (2011). Joint effects of dietary Vitamin D and sun exposure on breast cancer risk: Results from the French E3N cohort. *Cancer Epidemiology, Biomarkers, and Prevention, 20*(1), 187–198.

Erdfelder, E., Faul, F., & Buchner, A. (1996). GPOWER: A general power analysis program. *Behavior Research Methods, Instruments, and Computers, 28*(1), 1–11.

Erten, G. (⌐2016). TaqI, BsmI, and ApaI polymorphisms in the Vitamin D Receptor and genotype frequencies in female breast cancer and increase in the risk of nephrolithiasis. Retrieved from https://www.hindawi.com/journals/dm/2016/7475080/

Fayanju, O. M., Kraenzle, S., Drake, B. F., Oka, M., & Goodman, M. S. (2014). Perceived barriers to mammography among underserved women in a breas thealth center outreach program. *The American Journal of Surgery, 208*(3), 425–434. doi:10.1016/j.amjsurg.2014.03.005

Feng, Y., Stram, D. O., Rhie, S. K., Millikan, R. C., Ambrosone, C. B., John, E. M., . . . Haiman, C. (2014). A comprehensive examination of breast cancer risk loci in African American women. *Human Molecular Genetics, 23*(20), 5518–5526.doi:10.1093/hmg/ddu252

Freedman, M. L., Haiman, C. A., Patterson, N., McDonald, G. J., Tandon, A., Waliszewska, A., . . .Reich, D. (2006). Admixture mapping identifies 8q24 as a prostate cancer risk locus in African-American men. *Proceedings of the National Academy of Sciences of the United States of America, 103*(38), 14068–14073. doi:10.1073/pnas.0605832103

Fuhrman, B. J., Freedman, D. M., Bhatti, P., Doody, M. M., Fu, Y. P., Chang, S. C., . . .Sigurdson, A. J. (2013). Sunlight, polymorphisms of Vitamin D-related genes and risk of breast cancer. *Anticancer Research, 33*(2), 543-551.

Gallicchio, L., Helzlsouer, K. J., Chow, W. H., Freedman, D. M., Hankinson, S. E., Hartge, P., . . .Weinstein, S. J. (2015). Circulating 25-hydroxyVitamin D and the risk of rarer cancers: Design and methods of the Cohort Consortium Vitamin D Pooling Project of Rarer Cancers. *American Journal of Epidemiology, 172*(1), 10–20. doi:10.1093/aje/kwq116

Gnagnarella, P., Pasquali, E., Serrano, D., Raimondi, S., Disalvatore, D., & Gandini, S. (2014). Vitamin D Receptor polymorphism FokI and cancer risk: A comprehensive meta-analysis. *Carcinogenesis, 35*(9), 1913–1919. doi:10.1093/carcin/bgu150

Goodwin, P. J., Ennis, M., Pritchard, K. I., Koo, J.,& Hood, N. (2009).Prognostic effects of 25-hydroxyVitamin D Levels in early breast cancer. *Journal of Clinical Oncology, 27*(23), 3757–3763. doi:10.1200/JCO.2008.20.0725

Grant, W. B. (2013).An ecological study of cancer incidence and mortality rates in France with respect to latitude, an index for Vitamin D production. *Dermato-Endocrinology, 2*(2), 62–67.

Gudmundsson, J., Sulem, P., Manolescu, A., Amundadottir, L. T., Gudbjartsson, D., Helgason, A., . . . Stefansson, K. (2007). Genome-wide association study identifies a second prostate cancer susceptibility variant at 8q24. *Nature Genetics, 39*(5), 631–637. doi: 10.1038/ng1999

Gupta, A., Shridhar, K., & Dhillon, P. K. (2015). A review of breast cancer awareness among women in India: Cancer literate or awareness deficit? *Caucasian Journal of Cancer, 51*(14), 2058–2066. doi:10.1016/j.ejca.2015.07.008

Guy, M., Lowe, L. C., Bretherton-Watt, D., Mansi, J. L., Peckitt, C., Bliss, J., . . .V. Colston, K. W. (2004). Vitamin D Receptor gene polymorphisms and breast cancer risk. *Clinical Cancer Research 10*(16), 5472–5481. doi:10.1158/1078-0432.CCR-04-0206

Guy, M., Lowe, L. C., Bretherton-Watt, D., Mansi, J. L., Peckitt, C., Bliss, J., . . . Colston, K. W. (2013).BsmI but not FokI polymorphism of VDR gene is contributed in breast cancer. *Medical Oncology, 30*(1), 393. Retrieved from link.springer.com/content/pdf/10.1007/s12032-012-0393-7.pdf

Guyton, K. Z., Kensler, T. W., & Posner, G. H. (2003). Vitamin D and Vitamin Danalogs as cancer chemopreventive agents. *Nutrition Review, 61*(7), 227–38.

Haga, S. B., & LaPointe, N. M. A. (2013). The potential impact of pharmacogenetic testing on medication adherence. *The Pharmacogenomics Journal, 13*, 481–483. doi:10.1038/tpj.2013.33

Haiman, C. A., & Stram, D. O. (2015). Exploring genetic susceptibility to cancer in diverse populations. *Current Opinion in Genetics and Development, 20*(3), 330–335. doi:10.10 16/j.gde.2010.02.007

Ham, O. K. (2006). Factors affecting mammography behavior and intention among Korean women. *Oncology Nursing Forum, 33*(1), 113–119.

Harvie, M., Cohen, H., Mason, C., Mercer, T., Malik, R., Adams, J., . . . Howell, A. (2013). Adherence to a diet and weight loss intervention amongst women at increased risk of breast cancer. *Open Obesity Journal, 2*, 71–80.

Hung, M. (2015). *The behavioral impact of knowledge on breast cancer risk reduction.* (Walden University Doctoral dissertation).

Jaaskelainen, T., Ryhanen, S., Mahonen, A., De Luca, H. F.,&Maenpaa, P. H. (2010).Mechanism of action of superactiveVitamin Danalogs through regulated Receptor degradation. *Journal of Cell Biochemistry, 76*,548–558.

Jemal, A., Siegel, R., Ward, E., Hao, Y., Xu, J., Murray, T., & Thun, M. J. (2008). *Cancer statistics, 2008. CA: A Cancer Journal for Clinicians 58*(2),71–96.

John,E. M., Schwartz, G. G., Dreon, D. M., & Koo, J. (2011). Vitamin D and breast cancer: interpreting current evidence.doi:10.1186/bcr2846

Jones & Bartlett Learning. (2016) – Images for Health Belief Model. Retrieved from www.jblearning.com/samples/0763743836/

Jones, B. A., Reams, K., Calvocoressi, L., Dailey, A., Kasl, S. V., & Liston, N. M. (2007). Adequacy of communicating results from screening mammograms to African American and Caucasian women. *American Journal of Public Health,97*(3), 531–538. Retrieved from http://dx.doi.org/10.2105/AJPH.2005.076349

Katz, M. H. (2006). *Health programs in Bayview Hunter's Point and recommendations for improving the health of Bayview Hunter's Point residents.* Retrieved fromhttp://www. sfdph.org/dph/files/reports/StudiesData/BayviewHlthRpt09192006

Kemmis, C. M.,& Welsh, J. (2008). Mammary epithelial cell transformation is associated with deregulation of the Vitamin D pathway. *Journal of Cell Biochemistry, 105*(4), 980–988. doi: 10.1002/jcb.21896

Khokhar, A. (2009). Level of awareness regarding breast cancer and its screening amongst Indian teachers. *Asian Pacific Journal of Cancer Prevention, 10,* 247–250.

Knight, J.A., Lesosky, M., Barnett, H., Raboud, J.M., & Vieth, R. (2007). Vitamin D and reduced risk of breast cancer: A population-based case-control study. *Cancer Epidemiology, Biomarkers & Prevention,16*(3), 422–429. doi:10.1158/1055-9965.EPI-06-0865

Krishnan, A. V., & Feldman, D. (2011). Mechanisms of the anti-cancer and anti-inflammatory actions of Vitamin D. *Annual Review of Pharmacology and Toxicology,51,* 311–336.

Kulis, M., & Esteller, M. (2010). DNA methylation and cancer. *Advances in Genetics, 70,* 27-56. doi:10.1016/B978-0-12- 380866-0.60002-2

Kuper,H., Yang, L.,Sandin, S., Lof, M., Adami,H. O., & Weiderpass,E. (2009). Prospective study of solar exposure, dietary Vitamin D intake, and risk of breast cancer among middle-aged women. *Cancer Epidemiology, Biomarkers & Prevention,18*(9), 2558–2561.

La Forge, R. (2005). Aligning mind and body: Exploring the disciplines of mindful exercise. *ACSMs Health & Fitness Journal, 9,* 7–14.

Lee, J. H., Paul, S., Atalla, N., Thomas, P. E., Lin, X., Yang, I.,. . . Suh, N. (2008). Gemini Vitamin D analogues inhibit estrogen Receptor -positive and estrogen Receptor -negative mammary tumorigenesis without hypercalcemic toxicity. *Cancer Prevention Research, 1*(6), 476–484.

Lee,H., Kim, J., & Han, H. (2009). Do cultural factors predict mammography behavior among Korean immigrants?*Journal of Advanced Nursing, 65*(12): 2574–2584. doi: 10.11/j.1365-2648.2009.05155.x

Lemlem, S. B.,Sinishaw, W.,Hailu, M.,Abebe, M., & Aregay, A. (2011). Assessment of knowledge of breast cancer and screening methods among nurses in university hospitals in Addis Ababa, Ethiopia.doi:10.1155/2013/470981

Li, S. S.,Tseng, H. M., Yang,T. P., Liu, C. H., Teng, S. J., Huang, H.,. . . Tsai, J. H. (1999). Molecular characterization of germline mutations in the BRCA1 and BRCA2 genes from breast cancer families in Taiwan. *Human Genetics, 104*(3), 201–204.

Lin, F. H., Menton, U., Pett, M., Nail, L., Lee, S., & Mooney, K. (2008). Measuring breast cancer and mammography screening beliefs among Chinese-American immigrants. *Western Journal of Nursing Research, 30,* 853–868.

Lipsey, M.W., & Wilson, D.B. (1993).The efficacy of psychological, educational, and behavioral treatment: Confirmation from meta-analysis.*American Psychologist, 49*(12), 1181–1209.

Lu, D., Jing, L., & Zhang, S. (2016). Vitamin DReceptorpolymorphismand breast cancer risk: A meta-analysis. *Medicine (Baltimore), 95*(18), e3535. doi:10.1097/MD.0000000000003535.

Luo, S.,Guo, L.,Li, Y.,&Wang, S. (2014). Vitamin DReceptorgene ApaI polymorphism and breast cancer susceptibility: Ameta-analysis. *Tumour Biology, 35*(1),785–790. doi: 10.1007/s13277-013-1107-2.

Mamdouh, H. M.,El-Mansy, H., Kharboush, I. F., Ismail, H. M., Tawfik, M. M., El-Baky, M. A.,& El-Sharkawy, O. G. (2014). Barriers to breast cancer screening among a sample of Egyptian females. *Journal of Family and Community Medicine, 21*(2), 119–124. doi:10.4103/2230-8229.134771

Mangum, L. (2016). Identifying the beliefs and barriers to mammography in rural African American women. (Walden University Doctoral dissertation.)

Manolio, T. A. (2010). Genomewide association studies and assessment of the risk of disease. *The New England Journal of Medicine, 363*(2), 166–176.

Manolio, T. A., Brooks, L. D., & Collins, F. S. (2008). A HapMap harvest of insights into the genetics of common disease. *Journal of Clinical Investigation, 118*(5), 1590–1605. doi: 10.1172/JCI34772

McDonald-Mosley, R. (2016). *Planned Parenthood shares new survey data on women's knowledge and access to breast and cervical cancer screenings.* Retrieved from www.plannedparenthood.org/about-us/newsroom/press-releases/planned-parenthood-shares-new-survey-data-on-womens-knowledge-and-access-to-breast-and-cervical-cancer-screenings

McGee, S. A., Durham, D. D., Tse, C. K., &Millikan, R. C. (2014). *The Carolina Breast Cancer Study. Race and breast cancer subtypes.* Retrieved from http://cbcs.web.unc.edu/race-and-breast-cancer-subtypes/

McKay, J. D.,McCullough, M. L.,Ziegler, R. G.,Kraft, P., Saltzman, B. S.,Riboli, E., . . .Thun, M. J. (2009). Vitamin DReceptorpolymorphisms and breast cancer risk: Results from the National Cancer Institute Breast and Prostate Cancer Cohort Consortium. *Cancer Epidemiology, Biomarkers &Prevention,18*(1), 297–305. doi: 10.1158/1055-9965. EPI-08-0539

Mishra, D. K. (ʃ2013). Vitamin DReceptorGene Polymorphisms and Prognosis of Breast Cancer. Retrieved from journals.plos.org/plosone/article/file?id=10.1371/journal.pone.0057967&type...

Mishra, W., Sarkissyan, M., Chen, Z., Sarkissyan, S., Shang, X., Ong, M., . . .Vadgama, J. V. (2013). Vitamin DReceptorgene polymorphisms and prognosis of breast cancer among African-American and Hispanic women. *PLoS One, 8*(3),e57967. doi:10.1371/journal.pone.0057967

Mohr,S. B., Garland,C. F., Gorham,E. D., Grant,W. B.,& Garland, F. C. (2008). Relationship between low ultraviolet B irradiance and higher breast cancer risk in 107 countries. *Breast Journal, 14*(3), 255–260.doi: 10.1111/j.1524-4741.2008.00571

Nair, R., & Maseeh, A. (2012). Vitamin D: The "sunshine" vitamin. *Journal of Pharmacology and Pharmacotherapy, 3*(2),118–126. doi:10.4103/0976-500X.95506

Naqvi, A. A., Zehra, F., Ahmad, R., & Ahmad, N. (2016). *Developing a research instrument to document awareness, knowledge, and attitudes regarding breast cancer and early detection techniques for Pakistani women: The Breast Cancer Inventory (BCI).* Retrieved from www. mdpi.com/2079-9721/4/4/37/pdf

National Cancer Institute. (2015). Cancer health disparities. Retrieved fromwww.cancer.gov/about-nci/organization/crchd/cancer-health-disparitiesfact-sheet

National Cancer Institute. (2016). Breast Cancer Treatment. Journal of American Board of Family Medicine. Clinical Oncology 14 (5): 1730-6 doi:10.3122/jabfm.2009.01.070188

National Cancer Institute. (2017). Cancer causes and prevention. Retrieved fromwww.cancer.gov/about-cancer/causes-prevention/risk/diet/vitamin-d-fact-sheet.

Neff,R. T., Senter,L., &Salani, R. (2017). BRCAmutation in ovarian cancer: Testing, implications and treatment considerations. *Therapeutic Advances in Medical Oncology, 9*(8), 519–531. doi:10.1177/1758834017714993

Nelson, M. E, Rejeski, W.J., Blair, S.N., Duncan, P. W., Judge, J. O., King, A.C. . . . Castaneda-Sceppa, C. (2007). Physical activity and public health in older adults: Recommendation from the American College of Sports Medicine and the American Heart Association. *Medical Science Sports Exercise,39*(8), 1435–1445.

Nicholls, M. E. R. (2010). *Likert scales.* doi:10.1002/9780470479216.corpsy0508

Odusanya, O. O., & Tayo, O. O. (2001). Breast cancer knowledge, attitudes, and practices among nurses in Lagos, Nigeria. *Acta Oncologica, 40*(7), 844–848.

Oh, M. G., Han, M. A., Park, J., Ryu, S. Y., & Choi, S. W. (2015). The prevalence of Vitamin Ddeficiency among cancer survivors in a nationwide survey of the Korean population. *PLoS One, 10*(6), e0129901.doi.org/10.1371/journal.pone.0129901

Ohanuka, S. (2017). Assessing nurses' demographic cardiovascular risk factors and pharmacogenetic testing knowledge and acceptance. (Walden University Doctoral dissertation0.

Parsa, P., Kandiah, M., Zulkefli, N. A. M., & Rahman, H. A. (2008). Knowledge andbehavior regarding breast cancer screening among female teachers in Selangor, Malaysia. *Asian Pacific Journal of Cancer Prevention, 9*(2), 221–227.

Piazza, D., Foote, A., Holcombe, J., Harris, M. G., & Wright, P. (2007). The use of Roy's Adaptation

Model applied to a patient with breast cancer. Retrieved from https://onlinelibrary.wiley.com/doi/abs/10.1111/j.1365-2354.1992.tb00128.x

Peng, L., Xu, T., Long, T., & Zuo, H. (2016). Association between BRCA status and P53 status in breast cancer: A meta-analysis. *Medical Science Monitor, 22*, 1939–1945.doi:10.12659/MSM.896260

Rainville, C.,Khan, Y.,&Tisman, G. (2009). Triple negative breast cancer patients presenting with low serum Vitamin Dlevels: A case series.*Cases Journal,2*, 8390. doi:10.4076/1757-1626-2-8390

Ries, L. A. G., Eisner, M. P., Kosary, C. L., Hankey, B. F., Miller, B. A., Clegg, L., & Edwards, B. K. (Eds.). (2001). *SEER Cancer Statistics Review, 1973–1998*, National Cancer Institute,Bethesda, MD. Retrieved fromhttps://seer.cancer.gov/archive/csr/1973_1998/

Ristevska-Dimitrovska, G.,Filov, I.,Rajchanovska, D., Stefanovski, P., &Dejanova, B. (2015). Resilience and quality of life in breast cancer patients. *Open Access Macedonian Journal of Medical Sciences, 3*(4), 727–731.doi:10.3889/oamjms.2015.128

Roberts, M. C.,Weinberger, M.,Dusetzina, S. B., Dinan, M. A., Reeder-Hayes, K. E.,Troester, M. A.,. . . Wheeler, S. B. (2015). Racial variation in adjuvant chemotherapy initiation among breast cancer patients receiving oncotype DX testing. *Breast Cancer Research and Treatment, 153*(1), 191–200. doi:10.1007/s10549-015-3518-9

Rogers, C., & Keller, C. (2009). Roy's Adaptation Model to promote physical activity among sedentary older adults. *Geriatric Nursing, 30*(2 Suppl), 21–26. Retrieved from https://www.ncbi.nlm.nih.gov/pmc/articles/PMC2855388/doi:10.1016/j.gerinurse.2009.02.002

Rudestam, K. E.,& Newton, R. R. (2007).Surviving your dissertation: A comprehensive guide to content and process. New York, NY: Sage.

Sadler, G. R., Takahashi, M., Ko, C. M., & Nguyen, T. (2003). Japanese-American women: Behaviors and attitudes toward breast cancer education and screening. *Health Care for Women International, 24*, 18–26.

Sambanje, M. N., & Mafuvadze, B. (2012). Breast cancer knowledge and awareness among university students in Angola. *Pan African Medical Journal,11*, 70.

Shahbazi, S.,Alavi, S.,Majidzadeh,A. K.,Ghaffarpour, M.,Soleimani, A.,& Mahdian,R. (2016). BsmI but not FokI polymorphism of VDR gene is contributed in breast cancer. *Medical Oncology,30*(1), 393. doi:10.1007/s12032-012-0393-7

Shan, J. L., Dai, N.,Yang,X. Q.,Qian, C. Y., Yang, Z. Z.,Jin, F., . . . Wang, D.(2014). FokI polymorphism in Vitamin DReceptorgene and risk of breast canceramong Caucasian women. *Tumour Biology, 35*(4), 3503–3508. doi:10.1007/s13277-013-1462-z. Epub 2013 Dec 8.

Stangor, C. (2014). *Research methods for the behavioral sciences*. Chicago, IL: Cengage Learning.

Susan G. Komen (n.d.). *Komen for the cure.* (2015). Retrieved from ww5.komen.org/

Susan G. Komen. (n.d.). *Race for the cure.* ww5.komen.org/Breastcancer/Facts and Statistics.html

Susan G. Komen. (2017). *2018 Komen Dallas race for the cure.* Retrieved fromwww.info-komen. org/site/TR?fr_id=6940

Swami, S., Krishnan, A. V., Wang, J. Y., Jensen, K., Horst, R., Albertelli, M.A., & Feldman, D. (2012). Dietary Vitamin D3and 1, 25-dihydroxyvitamin D3(calcitriol) exhibit equivalent anticancer activity in mouse xenograft models of breast and prostate cancer. *Endocrinology, 153*(6), 2576–2587.

Trabert, B., Malone, K. E., Daling, J. R., Doody, D. R., Bernstein, L., Ursin, G., . . . Ostrander, E. A. Vitamin D Receptor polymorphisms and breast cancer risk in a large population-based case-control study of Caucasian and African-American women. *Breast Cancer Research 9*(6), R84. doi:10.1186/bcr1833

Uitterlinden, A. G., Fang, Y., van Meurs, J. B., Pols, H. A., & van Leeuwen, J. P. (2014).Genetics and biology of Vitamin D Receptor polymorphisms. *Gene, 338*(2):143–156.

U. S. Department of Health and Human Services. *Healthy people 2010.*Retrieved fromhttps:// www.cdc.gov/nchs/healthy_people/hp2010.htm

U. S. National Breast Cancer Foundation. (2015). *Service King, National Breast Cancer Foundation partner in early detection awareness.* Retrieved from nationalbreastcancer.org/press-release/2015/10/01/service-king-national-breast-cancer-foundation-partner-in-early-detection-awareness

Uwuseba, L. (2010). Knowledge, attitudes, and behaviors of African American women regarding breast cancer screening. (Walden University Doctoral dissertation)

Wang, J., He, Q., Shao, Y., Ji, M., & Bao, W. (2013). Associations between Vitamin D Receptor polymorphisms and breast cancer risk. *Tumour Biology, 34*(6):3823–3830. doi:10.1007/ s13277-013-0967-9

Wang, W., Hsu, S., Wang, J., Huang, L., & Hsu, W. (2014). Survey of breast cancer mammography screening behaviors in Eastern Taiwan based on a health belief model. *The Kaohsiung Journal of Medical Sciences, 30*(8), 422–427.doi.org/10.1016/j.kjms.2014.04.007

Witte, K. (1992). Putting the fear back into fear appeals: The extended parallel process model. *Communication Monographs,59*(4), 329–349. Retrieved from https://www.tandfonline. com/doi/abs/10.1080/03637759209376276

Witte, K. (1994). Fear control and danger control: A test of the extended parallel process model (EPPM).*Communication Monographs,61*(2), 113–134. Retrieved from https://www. tandfonline.com/doi/abs/10.1080/03637759409376328

World Health Organization. (2013). *Women's health.* Retrieved from http://www.who.int/ news-room/fact-sheets/detail/women-s-health

Wu, T. Y., West, B., Chen, Y. W., &Hergert, C. (2005). Health beliefs and practices related to breast cancer screening in Filipino, Chinese, and Asian-Indian Women. *Cancer Detection and Prevention, 30*(1), 58–66.

Wynstra, N. A. (2011). *Breast cancer: Selected legal issues.* Retrievedfromhttp://onlinelibrary. wiley.com/doi/10.1002/cncr.2820741339/pdf

Xu, H.,Li, S.,Qiu, J.Q.,Gao, X.L.,Zhang, P.,&Yang, Y.X, (2013). The VDR Gene FokI polymorphism and ovarian cancer risk. *Tumour Biology, 34*(6):3309–3316.

Yang,L., Lof, M., Veierød, M. B., Sandin,S., Adami,H. O., &Weiderpass,E. (2011).Ultraviolet exposure and mortality among women in Sweden. *Cancer Epidemiology, Biomarkers & Prevention, 20*(4), 683–690. doi:10.1158/1055-9965.EPI-10-0982

Young-McCaughan, S., Arzola, T. M., Leclerc, K. M., Shry, E. A., Sheffler, R. L., Nowlin, M. U., & Dramiga, S. A. (2007). Exercise tolerance 18-months following participation in an exercise program for patients treated for cancer.*Oncology Nursing Forum, 34*(1), 189.

Zhang,K.,& Song, L. (2014). Association between Vitamin DReceptorgenepolymorphisms and breast cancer risk: A meta-analysis of 39 studies. *PLoS One, 9*(4), e96125.doi.org/10.1371/journal.pone.0096125

Zhang, X., Han, X., Dang, Y., Meng, F., Guo, X.,& Lin, J. (2016). User acceptance of mobile health services from users' perspectives: The role of self-efficacy and response-efficacy in technology acceptance. *Informatics for Health and Social Care, 42*(2), 194–206.doi:10.1080/17538157.2016.1200053

Appendix A:Permission to Use Self-Administered Web-Based Survey Material

AMERICAN ASSOCIATION FOR CANCER RESEARCH LICENSE
TERMS AND CONDITIONS

Jul 31, 2017

This Agreement between Ejike R. Egwuekwe ("You") and American Association for Cancer Research ("American Association for Cancer Research") consists of your license details and the terms and conditions provided by American Association for Cancer Research and Copyright Clearance Center.

License Number	4159571072378
License date	Jul 31, 2017
Licensed Content Publisher	American Association for Cancer Research
Licensed Content Publication	Cancer Research
Licensed Content Title	Self-administered, web-based screening of family history of cancer as a method to select appropriate patients for genetic assessment.
Licensed Content Author	LS Acheson,A Lynn,GL Wiesner
Licensed Content Date	Jan 15, 2009
Licensed Content Volume	69
Licensed Content Issue	2 Supplement
Type of Use	Thesis/Dissertation

Appendix B: Breast Cancer Survey

1. Which of the following is(are) the problem(s) I have, which may prevent me from direct exposure to sunlight?
   a. I do not like direct exposure to sunlight
   b. I have a medical problem that preventsme from direct exposure to sunlight
   c. My religion or culture prevents me from having direct exposure to sunlight
   d. I do not have problems with direct exposure to sunlight

2. Which of the following are your sources of vitamin D? Please select all that apply.
   a. Exposure to sunlight
   b. Vitamin Ddietary supplements
   c. Vitamin Danalogs
   d. I am allergic to either Vitamin Dsupplements or analogs

3. Which of the following is not a risk factor for breast cancer?
   a. Early menstrual flow or menarche
   b. Late menopause
   c. Poor Vitamin D intake
   d. Balanced diet

4. Mammograms can help detect breast cancer at early stage: TrueorFalse

5. Breast self-exams are necessary for detecting breast lumps: TrueorFalse

6. Intake of Vitamin Dcan help reduce breast cancer incidence rate: TrueorFalse

7. The older a woman gets, the higher her chances of contracting breast cancer: TrueorFalse

8. In America, the lifetime risk of contracting breast cancer is one in:
   a. 10
   b. 8
   c. 6
   d. 4

Appendix C: Knowledge of Vitamin D Receptor Gene Polymorphisms

QUESTIONNAIRE:
Breast cancer screening practices knowledge, attitudes and practice of breast cancer screening among women in Dallas, Houston, and San Antonio, Texas.

This study is being conducted on breast cancer risk factors and breast cancer prevention. Your responses will be kept confidential. Your honest answer will be appreciated. Participation is not compulsory. You are at liberty to withdraw from the study at any time, without being asked your reason for doing so. Thanks for responding and for your time.

SECTION A: SOCIODEMOGRAPHICS & CHARACTERISTICS

1. Age at last birthday (years): _____
2. Marital status – Please Select One:
(1) Single/Never married (2) Married/Cohabiting (3) Separated/Divorced/Widowed
3. Occupation: _____ (Categorized into formal, Informal and unemployed)
4. Race: (1) Black (2) White (3) Other (please specify) _____
4. Highest level of education: (1) Less than High School (2) Completed High School or GED (3) Some college, but did not complete (4) Completed 4 years of college. (5) Graduate/Professional degrees). _____

SECTION B: KNOWLEDGE OF VITAMIN D RECEPTOR GENE POLYMORPHISMS AND BREAST CANCER

5. Do you know about breast cancer? (1) Yes (2) No
6. Do you have breast cancer? (1) Yes (2) No
7. Has any member of your family been diagnosed of breast cancer? (1) Yes (2) No
8. If answer to the question above is yes, what is her relationship to you? (1) Mother (2) Aunt (3) Sister (4) Cousin (5) Others (specify)_____
9. To what extent do you know about Vitamin D Receptor gene polymorphisms and the association with breast cancer? (1) I don't (2) To a low extent (3) To a large extent (4) To a very large extent.
10. If you (or any member of your family had been clinically diagnosed with breast cancer), were you (or the family member also diagnosed with low serum Vitamin D? (1) Yes (2) No
11. If you (or any member of your family had been clinically diagnosed with breast cancer), was the breast cancer associated with low vitamin D (or Vitamin D Receptor gene polymorphisms? (1) Yes (2) No

Questions 10 & 11:

10. Have you or any member of your family been diagnosed with low serum vitamin D?

    1. [Never] 2. [Once] 3. [On two Occasions] 4. [On more than two occasions]

11. Have you or any member of your family had a clinical case of vitamin D Receptor gene polymorphisms?

    1. [Never] 2. [Once] 3. [On two Occasions] 4. [On more than two occasions]

12. Based on what you know of VDR polymorphisms on breast cancer risks, will you use mammograms, and enroll in breast cancer risk-reduction programs to reduce chances of breast cancer?

(1) Yes (2) No

If yes, why? (Please explain) _____

If no, why? (Please explain) _____

- Note: If you or your family member had been diagnosed with breast cancer, and you do not know (or do not understand) anything about Vitamin D Receptor polymorphism and its association with breast cancer risk, please ask your Doctor or Nurse, before completing the portion of the questionnaire about Vitamin D Receptor gene polymorphisms. Thank you.

Appendix D: Survey of Participants' Response Efficacy

The following are examples of the types of questions used in the assessment questionnaire for response efficacy.

On a scale of 1 to 5, please indicate your feeling and personal motivation on each of the following Likert Scale questions.

1. Exposure to Vitamin Dcan be helpful in reducing my risk of breast cancer.
   a. Strongly agree
   b. Agree
   c. Neither agree nor disagree
   d. Disagree
   e. Strongly disagree

2. Vitamin DReceptorpolymorphisms can increase chances of getting breast cancer.
   a. Strongly agree
   b. Agree
   c. Neither agree nor disagree
   d. Disagree
   e. Strongly disagree

3. Genetic testing can help me identify any risk factors for breast cancer.
   a. Strongly agree
   b. Agree
   c. Neither agree nor disagree
   d. Disagree
   e. Strongly disagree

Index

Printed in the United States
By Bookmasters